Every Patient You See

Every Patient You See

Loving Your Life In General Practice

Dr David Ringelblum

Every Patient You See: Loving Your Life In General Practice

First published in Australia by David Ringelblum.

Cover by Monique Bendel.

Cataloguing
ISBN (paperback) 978-1-7645881-0-2
ISBN (Kindle) 978-1-7645881-1-9
ISBN (audiobook) 978-1-7645881-2-6

BISAC code MED029000 **MEDICAL**/Family & General practice

NATIONAL LIBRARY OF AUSTRALIA
A catalogue record for this book is available from the National Library of Australia

DEDICATION

To my parents – for all that they taught me
To my teachers – for all that they taught me
To my colleagues – for all that they taught me
To my registrars – for all that they taught me
 and abovc all
To my patients – for all that they taught me

און פאַר די וואָס באַשײַנען מײַן לעבן.

I would like to acknowledge the Boonwurrung and Wurundjeri/Woiwurrung people of the Kulin nation, the traditional custodians of the lands on which this book was written. I remain dismayed at the unacceptable gap which exists in the life expectancy, health outcomes and wellness between Aboriginal and Torres Strait Islander people and the rest of the Australian community.
We can, we must, do better.

Every patient you see is a lesson in much more than the malady from which he suffers.

Dr William Osler, The Student Life, 1914

Contents

Preface

What this book is not:

There are many, many books that will teach you the clinical aspects of medicine. This isn't one of them.
As introductory texts to taking a history and doing a physical examination, Macleod's *Clinical Examination* and Talley and O'Connor's *Clinical Examination* are both excellent primers.

If you want to learn how to structure a general practice consultation, then I recommend you start with Ron Roth and Julie Willem's seminal article in the *Australian Journal of General Practice* (AJGP) 51:5 pp 310-315. Every general practitioner (GP) from first day registrar to those about to retire can benefit from this outline.

https://www1.racgp.org.au/ajgp/2022/may/teaching-the-art-of-general-practice-consultation

Simon Morgan et al have written two other pieces which help outline a consulting schema for registrars. The first can be found in *Australian Family Physician* (AFP) 43:9 pp 645-648

RACGP - Starting off in gp – consultation tips for new GP registrars

This was followed up by additional material in AJGP 53:12 pp 916-920.

https://www1.racgp.org.au/getattachment/7922a46a-57b4-43b9-b638-072a9b50f2c8/Consultation-skill-tips-for-new-general-practice-r.aspx

These articles teach not just how to structure a consultation, but how to build one.

What this book is:

My hope is that this book will help you cultivate great consultations, close relationships and a thriving practice. And help you fall in love with being a GP.

It evolved along two separate pathways.

The first was through reflecting on the many mistakes I have made through the course of more than 35 years as a GP. Nearly all of that time has been in the same practice, though we are now in our third building, having moved from a house to a shopping centre to a purpose-built 31-room clinic.

Though I don't live there, I feel very connected to the suburb where I work. I've watched it grow, evolve, age. There are shopping centres that didn't exist when I started; the bursting at the seams primary schools are now back to a manageable size. When I joined, the suburb was basically new babies and their parents. Now the children I cared for in those first years are grown, and their parents are late middle age with chronic illnesses replacing child-rearing stresses.

My babies are having babies. Many of them however can't afford to live in the area where they grew up, and move to outer suburbs where land and housing is cheaper. Still, a remarkably complimentary number keep coming to see me. "Why are you travelling 30 minutes with a sick baby in the back of the car?" I ask them. And many reply "Because you looked after me when I was a baby, and I don't trust anyone else to look after mine."

I sometimes call myself a Grand-Doctor!

I certainly don't mean grand in the sense of better. But caring for three and four generations of the same family is a grand feeling, and perhaps gives you the status of somebody important in the stories members of a family tell each other.

During that time I've made just about every mistake known to medical-kind. I've hurt people physically, emotionally and iatrogenically. But I hope, by reflecting honestly, I've rarely made the same mistake multiple times. I would love you to avoid the mistakes I made; and your patients to benefit from the mistakes my patients suffered at my hands.

At the same time, I've done enough right to have a successful practice, loyal long-standing patients, and I hope a reputation of some honour in my neighbourhood.

So this book tells the story of how to become and what it means to be deeply entrenched as a general practitioner in the lives of individuals, families and a community.

The second pathway which led to this book has been through more than 25 years as a GP supervisor, during which time I've had the privilege and pleasure of mentoring around 100 registrars. Every registrar is different – they come to our practice with different personalities, experience, confidence, learning styles, values and ambitions. Hence, the process of teaching, leading, mentoring and supervising them requires thinking anew and with fresh eyes about precisely what to teach and how I will do so in a way that resonates with each individual.

One of my favourite teaching tools, valuable for nearly every registrar, is the sit-in tute, where I sit in a corner of the room, usually behind the patient so I remain out of eye-sight, and simply observe the consultation.

Once the patient has left the room, the registrar and I spend time reviewing the consultation. What went well? What could be better? What needs to be worked on?

Some of that discussion is based around the science of medicine, but very often we end up focussing on the philosophy of general practice and the art of the consultation.

The joy of general practice is that each person is different, yet humans are all the same. The same can be said of registrars. And so, over time, a collection of common teaching points evolved. These morphed into a set of sayings and aphorisms that I hope encapsulate some of the essence of good general practice.

I have no doubt that any thoughtful doctor develops these or their own similar set of rules over time. I don't claim special authority to proclaim these. Starting off in general practice can be scary, but nearly everyone gets there in the end, and most GPs do a fine job. So will you!

I do however hope that by confessing the mistakes I've made and relating the shortcomings I've seen in registrars you will learn more quickly than by making every mistake yourself. My intent is that reading this will accelerate your comfort to be alone in a consultation room with someone who has come to you in need, and hopefully this book will make the process a little less traumatic for you and for your patients.

The hallmark of general practice is continuity of care. Most specialists focus on one body part, one body system or one patient demographic. And those who deal with the undifferentiated patient – emergency physicians, home visiting locums – deal with one problem, one patient, one time.

But ***General practice, first and foremost, is about relationships with patients over time.***

The length, breadth and depth of a relationship with a patient is the greatest tool that a GP can have. It has diagnostic value, therapeutic value and human value.

A great general practice training term is one where you build relationships with patients. It's a taste of the career that lies just ahead of you.

~~~

The lessons stated here developed over decades and in the teaching of many registrars. Sometimes I say the same thing in different ways because different people need different words to speak to them meaningfully. I trust you can find something in here that speaks to you, and will forgive any repetition.

On the other hand, the reader may be frustrated that some of these rules contradict each other. It is the nature of aphorisms to do so – 'Actions speak louder than words', yet 'The pen is mightier than the sword'; 'Many hands make light work' but "Too many cooks spoil the broth.'

I have no answer other than to say that you must think for yourself which rules to apply when. They are merely suggestions – not commandments.

At the same time, please don't read it all in one sitting. In fact, **I encourage you to read no more than one chapter a day**, and then reflect on it in your following day's practice before moving on to the next chapter. Dip in and out, and perhaps re-read a relevant chapter if you have a difficult consultation. Maybe there is a clue somewhere about how it might have gone better.
~~~

As a general rule, I've tried to order the chapters from early Registrar to early Fellow. Everyone learns at a different pace and in a different order, but the intent is that the more basic lessons are up front and the more subtle ones later.

~~~

Some of what you read here is conventional medical or general practice wisdom. Some of it, I hope, is fresh. I know that I say some things that are out of fashion, some I think are ahead of fashion and some are perhaps just provocative. I do so to stimulate thinking, discussion and debate. Analysing and rejecting these ideas will be far more useful for your learning and growing than just accepting and rehashing them.

Above all, I am aware that any saying, adage or aphorism is a generalisation and therefore automatically an oversimplification. But general practice is about complexity. So, take none of what you read as absolute truth – merely suggestions for consideration.

More importantly, please think about how to apply and extend these thoughts to other situations. I hope that you find them applicable in multiple instances and not just those scenarios that I use as illustrations.

If you are a registrar, your practice supervisors will have their own rules. Listen carefully! They developed them for a reason, and in the particular setting of their practice. I would love to hear their aphorisms and would be grateful if you send them to me, with attribution. And if you develop your own, please be in touch.

If you are a supervisor or an experienced GP, you might think some or much of what I write is completely wrong! I look forward to hearing why you disagree with these rules or my musings, and any of your own that you would like to add. Please send me feedback! We only get better by learning from others. I can be reached at **everypatientyousee@gmail.com**.

~~~

A note on attribution. There is a Talmudic notion that when we quote the words of our teachers in their name, their lips move in the grave. My students find this unnerving, but I love the idea that as long as we quote a person, and not just a saying, that person lives on. I have therefore specifically named all those whose words I quote where I remember from whom I first heard them, and where I have been able to receive permission.

If any reader feels that I have quoted them without attribution, I apologise. We have either developed our ideas independently and in parallel, or I have plagiarised subconsciously and unwittingly. Please contact me to reprimand!

~~~

A final word to any of my patients reading this book. It is largely based on the mistakes I have made on you and the consultations I have witnessed with you. Though certain case histories are narrated, I assure you names, ages, genders and medical details have been changed enough to hide all identifying features. You might think you recognize yourself – but in any event no-one else will, and chances are it isn't even you.
~~~

A note for non-Australian readers

One of the reasons I chose to do medicine is that it was a "transportable profession". Regardless of where I would end up working, human physiology, pathology, psychology and nature would be largely the same. People are people wherever they live! And so I trust that the messages of this book will translate to wherever the reader is located.

The same however cannot be said for terminology, let alone the process of becoming a GP, and even less for the health care systems in which we each operate. This might lead to some confusion around terms or references in the chapters that follow. Allow me then to provide a very brief overview of becoming and being a GP in Australia.

I mostly use the term general practitioner or GP. This is the equivalent of family physician and largely overlaps with primary care practitioner or primary care physician, though my understanding is that the latter tend towards adult medicine rather than paediatrics and do less gynaecology and procedural medicine than an Australian GP might take on.

To become a GP in Australia involves a five-year undergraduate or four-year postgraduate medical degree. Success there results in a (now two-year) hospital-based internship with rotations in medical, surgical and emergency medicine terms as well as elective subspecialty rotations.

After at least two years in hospital - often more - those who wish to specialise in general practice apply to become registrars in the Royal Australian College of General Practitioners (RACGP) or the Australian College of Rural and Remote Medicine (ACCRM) for a two year program involving at least three six-month supervised general practice terms and one extended skills term which may involve further general practice or may be a term of obstetrics, skin cancer medicine, palliative care, sexual health, paediatrics etc. ACRRM require most of this training in regional or remote practices as well as an additional year of higher skills in surgery, obstetrics, anaesthetics or the like.

The training is a combination of lectures and tutorials provided by the training program, and hands-on education within the practice by experienced GP supervisors. These might be called teachers, trainers, mentors or educators in different contexts. Education includes formal and informal case discussion, didactic tutorials, demonstrating and then observing consultations, procedural skills and general philosophical chit-chat about a career in general practice.

Once training is completed and exams are passed, the newly Fellowed GP obtains a Medicare provider number entitling them and their patients to government contributions for medical care, and can then set up an independent practice, though is more likely to join an established private clinic which is either doctor or corporate owned. GPs are the centrepiece of the Australian health care system and patients generally will not see any specialist without having seen a GP who arranges suitable referral. Without the referral there is minimal government reimbursement for visits to specialists.

This means that the bulk of healthcare occurs in general practice clinics, because only if the GP feels unable to provide the procedural service or out of their medical knowledge depth do they send a patient to a specialist for opinion or management. In turn, this means GPs see most patients for most things most of the time.

Most general practice in Australia is private, though that may not involve out of pocket costs. GPs are free to charge whatever fee they wish. Through a universal health insurance scheme called Medicare, the government reimburses the patient a set fee depending on the time, complexity and procedure for each visit. The GP might agree to accept that fee as payment in full, in which case they directly bill the government (often called bulk-billing) and in return there is a small bonus incentive payment which the government hopes will encourage bulk-billing and therefore eliminate out of pocket costs to the public for healthcare. Market forces mean that many GPs bulkbill all or at least some of their patients. Over time the Medicare rebate/bulkbill payment has significantly fallen behind inflation and general cost of living. As a result, GPs have tended lately to charge private fees more often, often 50-100% more than the rebated amount, leaving patients with out-of-pocket gaps.

By contrast, nearly all specialists charge private fees (with a Medicare rebate to the patient if there is a valid referral.) In most cases, if patients cannot pay for private specialist visits or prefer not to, they can be referred - sometimes with a long waiting list – to a public hospital for free outpatient care.

The financial arrangements for hospital in-patient care are beyond this brief summary and largely not relevant to a discussion of general practice, which very rarely involves in-patient management, except in some rural settings.

Prologue

When I worked in ED …
I would tell patients to review with their GP.

But now I'm the GP …
and they're coming to see me …

My panic-stricken registrar,
2 weeks into first term of general practice.

CHAPTER 1

The Prime Directive

My first registrar experience of general practice was such a delight that I was overjoyed when the clinic asked me to moonlight two or three nights a week after I finished my term and went on to my next rotation in geriatrics. There were no Medicare provider number restrictions in those days, and so at some point in the afternoon I would call the clinic to ask how busy they were. If they needed my help seeing the winter overflow cohort of coughs, colds and otitis media, I would leave the hospital at 5pm, arrive at 6pm and see patients for two hours. Not only that – they paid me for it!

Truth be told, I enjoyed myself so much doing general practice, at that practice, that I honestly would have done it unpaid. To receive the magnificent sum of $25 per hour for doing something I loved was an amazing bonus!

One patient that I saw stands out in my memory, though it was more than 35 years ago. A young man, in his mid-20s, presented with severe headaches of recent onset. They were variable in severity, though a background headache was constant, and being debilitating enough to convince a young man to attend the GP was red flag enough.

At this point I had been a doctor for barely 18 months. I knew that I knew very little. I also knew that I was expected to know a lot. And I knew that being about the same age as this patient didn't make him trust more that I knew what I was doing.

Worst of all - I really had no idea where to go next. I figured that just asking more questions would make me look incompetent, (see Chapter 11 for why that was a mistake!) so I asked him to sit up on the bed and started the examination. At least I could look professional!

As one does in all the TV shows, I started by taking his pulse. Except that I couldn't find it. I moved my fingers proximally and distally, medially and laterally. I knew where the radial artery was MEANT to be... It just wasn't presenting itself to me.

This was mortifying! How incompetent a doctor was I – and would I appear to be – if I couldn't even find a pulse? But I had an out. I would take his blood pressure and count his pulse that way. So, I wrapped the manual BP cuff (no automated machines in those days!) around his arm and started listening for a brachial pulse. Except that I couldn't hear anything there either.

Humiliated, I reached for his other arm. And there to my relief was a perfectly normal, regular pulse and on examination, a perfectly normal blood pressure. His neurological exam – to whatever degree I performed it – was quite unremarkable, and his cardiovascular exam was completely normal.

I don't recall what tests I sent him for to stall for time, but I did ask him to return a week later for review. This he dutifully did, while I checked off all his normal results. A brain CT followed a week after that. And at each visit, with increasing curiosity, I kept rechecking to see if his pulse or blood pressure had somehow miraculously reappeared – or perhaps not so much magically, but as a result of my incompetence receding with a few extra days of clinical experience.

At some point, I mentioned this problem to the registrar overseeing me on my day-job geriatrics rotation. He had recently passed his physician's fellowship examination, and his head was stuffed full of knowledge of every conceivable rarity. Not wanting to display my ignorance, I presented it as a general practice curiosity rather than a desperate cry for diagnostic help.

Rather offhand he mentioned a long list of differential diagnoses, many of which were conditions I had never heard of or had only the barest recollection of from my (rather unsuccessful) final year studies. "Unilateral absent pulses" he opined, "suggest a vasculitis, probably a giant cell arteritis. Consider polyarteritis nodosa and Takayasu's disease!".

With some delight – now that I had a possible diagnosis that would explain my examination struggles, as well as provide me with kudos within the practice for finding the zebra disease – I rang the patient and asked him to come back the following week when I would next be in the clinic, so we could investigate just what was going on.

To my disappointment he didn't attend. I was frustrated – here I was excitedly sitting on a wonder-diagnosis, and he wouldn't do his part to allow that to happen. How inconsiderate!

So, a week later, I rang him again, a little miffed at his lack of interest when I was doing everything I could to get to the bottom of this diagnostic dilemma. With completely unjustified arrogance I asked him why he hadn't attended. His reply floored me, shamed me and remains embedded in my heart and brain:

"Because you've not done anything about my headaches."

The most valuable lesson I have ever learned in general practice, and which is the essence of every single consultation:

You have to deal with the patient's agenda, before you deal with your own.

This doesn't mean that you only address the patient's issues; or that you ignore, suppress or defer critical issues that you uncover along the way. Raise those issues, explain why they matter, help reshape the patient's agenda so it aligns with yours. But if you have items that you wish to deal with which are not central to the patient's presentation, make sure you have at least clearly acknowledged the latter fully, and explain to the patient's satisfaction why you are dealing with matters that were not the patient's priority when he walked through your door.

The vast majority of failed consultations, patient complaints, poor Google reviews, requests for transfer of medical records, referrals to the medical board and general patient-doctor frustration are a result of failing to respect this rule. If this is the only thing that you get out of this book, I will be satisfied.

CHAPTER 2

Two Is Better Than One

What do patients most want from their GP? Clearly, they want a capable, knowledgeable doctor. But patients are notoriously poor judges of medical skills. What they are expert at is judging bedside manner. What patients want is someone who makes them feel heard, understood and cared for.

It is easy for doctors to be dismissive of bedside manner as a clinical skill, but I will argue that it is among the most important. Because no matter how brilliant you are, unless the patient is sitting in front of you, you don't have the opportunity to put that knowledge, skill, technique, experience, perspective and wisdom to use.

Until a patient feels that you have their best interests at heart, they have no reason to expose their heart to you, to extend to you their time, their money, their vulnerability, their problem. Until you show that you respect the gift they have brought you – their trust that you can help them – they have no reason to come to see you.

Which is why:

Your primary duty at any consultation is to get another one.

In case it needs emphasising, I do not by this mean overservicing, unnecessary reviews or recalling a patient without good clinical cause.

A case in point: a new patient came to see me. As is routine, I asked why he was attending us rather than his previous GP, who happened to be quite local. He explained that the other doctor didn't run an appointment system, always had a full waiting room and kept him waiting excessively long.

Aside simple hypertension he had no other particular health concerns. His blood pressure was well controlled, and apart from arranging a lipid and diabetes screen, I didn't feel it was necessary to do much else at that visit. I wrote a repeat script and handed it to him with a smile.

"When would you like to see me again?" he asked. I explained the script would cover six months and provided the blood results came back normal, he could simply return in half a year.

"Oh?" he said half hesitantly, half disapprovingly. "Dr Smith checks my blood pressure *every* month."

There were several lessons I took from that encounter. Here was a patient willing to undertake the inconvenience, if not cost, of monthly visits to his GP, not for clinical need, but simply because his doctor asked him to do so. He didn't know that monthly BP checks added nothing to his health. But he knew that here was a doctor interested enough in his well-being as to want to see him monthly, despite his obviously busy schedule and full waiting room. (Of course, monthly BP checks may well have explained why the waiting room was so full!)

The same GP was also known to review all children with viral infections daily for one week, "just to make sure that they haven't developed any complications." When doctors like me protested that nearly all children will make an uncomplicated recovery and that there was no need for review unless additional symptoms developed, some parents would respond that Dr Smith was showing himself to be a caring doctor. Unspoken was perhaps that this was in contrast to my cavalier attitude.

So, on the one hand, we have patients with unstable diabetes, profound depression or uncontrolled blood pressure whom we cannot convince to return for regular review despite our significant concern for their short and long term welfare, and on the other hand, some patients and doctors reach a symbiotic understanding that they will see each other as often as necessary and perhaps as often as possible.

Why the difference? Because the latter group of patients feel those doctors are providing them something personal – their care, concern, devotion, dedication. It is not about their medical skills – it is about the patients' perception of the doctors' offering.

There are doctors (or naturopaths, iridologists and rain drop therapists) who may lack our clinical knowledge and skills but have greater capacity to convince patients that they care. In the battle to engage with patients – they will win. The responsibility therefore lies with us to convince patients, through our bedside manner, of both the health and emotional value of returning to see us.

CHAPTER 3

Shakespeare Was Wrong

A few weeks into my first preclinical year of university medical training, the lecturer in Social and Preventative Health spoke about the desensitising effect of the medical course.

"You are all enthusiastic, idealistic and committed to caring for people. But by the time you reach fourth year (the first year of clinical school), you will no longer speak about "Mrs Jones, the mother of three who bakes amazing birthday cakes, who came in last night with abdominal pain", but of "the gall bladder on the fourth floor."

I took that foreshadowing seriously and swore that I would never become that medical student or doctor. I would never stop thinking of patients as people, rather than just the vector of something.

But of course, I did.

There may be lots of valid reasons why patients may be described only in clinical terms. Privacy, in particular, means that identifying patients by name may release personal details to a wider audience than intended. When scores of clinicians attend a Grand Round, the primary point is medical education, not clinical care for that particular patient. Presenting identifying details doesn't benefit their interests but might cause harm.

When solo general practice was the professional norm, of course GPs knew each of their patients by name. As practices have enlarged, it becomes less likely that anyone, even long-standing principals, will know everyone in the practice.

This has been compounded by the trend towards GPs working part-time. The less time a GP spends in a practice, the less she or he will meet the broad gamut of patients who attend. Subspecialisation and demographic stratification also narrow the encounters that GPs have within a practice, let alone across the community.

The "bio-psycho-social model of illness" evolved for good reason. Health has many facets, determinants and factors.

Synonyms for general practice like family medicine or community practice acknowledge this, and we do have responsibilities to public health (and to the public purse) beyond our consulting room. But our primary work begins with deeply knowing the patient in front of us.

In General Practice, every patient has a name.

A corridor consultation with your supervisor beginning with "I've got a 21-year-old woman with me who is incredibly anxious", is quite different from "I'm seeing Tina Henderson. She's a 21-year-old woman who is incredibly anxious". Your supervisor might know that Tina is the daughter of Bob, who lost his brother to a degenerative disease; or that Tina's sister has had six miscarriages. They might immediately home in on at least one possible cause for the anxiety. With TV-doctor sleuth-like accuracy, you can work into the consultation a key question "Are you trying to get pregnant?"

Knowing that family history isn't just a routine question to be ticked off a list but is actually a key determinant of both the physical and mental health of our patients, leads to understanding that exploring family history, and the effect of family history, gives us diagnostic clues and management power.

In *Romeo and Juliet,* Shakespeare dismissively asks "What's in a name?" The answer, in fact, is identity. Every patient is an individual. Unless we know the patient – and identify them by name – we can't begin to deal with their individual needs.

CHAPTER 4

Cigarettes And Freddo Frogs

Having told you how important it is to be open to and responsive to what a patient wants, I am now going to tell you that it is far from the most important thing that you will do.

Certainly, you need to listen - and show you have heard - what a patient wants. Nobody knows better than the patient what they *think* they want. But in fact, patients are often not the best judge of what they really want, or rather what they really need.

A simple example: a patient comes in wanting repeat scripts for his 3-month overseas holiday. He wants medications. What he doesn't know is that:

- He needs a special Regulation 24 script to collect three months medication at one time
- He may need a letter from his GP to show Border Control when leaving Australia or entering another country explaining why he is carrying large quantities of medication
- He may need a health summary to carry with him, in case he needs medical help whilst overseas
- He may need travel vaccinations, water purifying tablets, travel sickness or altitude sickness medications, insecticide with DEET, help dealing with timing medication doses whilst crossing time zones, help obtaining adequate travel insurance etc etc

A request for repeat scripts tagged on to the end of a consultation is what the patient wants. Your job is to identify his needs - and hopefully in a timely manner, so that you can address those needs during that initial consultation or ensure the patient's understanding as to why you require him to come back, perhaps more than once.

This ultimately means teaching the patient why what he initially *thought* he wanted, and what he *really* wants (ie what you know he *needs*) is often far from the same thing.

A patient may want benzodiazapines. What he needs is better sleep. He may want opiates. What he needs is to be able to function fully despite pain rather than without pain. He may want a referral to a dermatologist. What he needs is a skin check or excision that you can perform, faster, cheaper and just as well. He may want the blood tests his naturopath recommended you order. What he needs is to understand the poor predictive value of most tests for screening.

If you've ever been shopping with a 3-year-old, the distinction will be very clear. "I have to have a chocolate frog ... I have to! I have to!!" No, you don't have to. You just really want it.

It's an analogy I often use with smokers describing the habit of smoking after meals or with a coffee in one hand and a cigarette in the other – you may desperately want a cancer-stick but that doesn't mean that you need one.

What does the patient want? What does the patient need?

Distinguishing those two, and reconciling them, is a key task. Once a patient develops a trust in you, he will be much more willing to come to you with a problem, and have you guide him to the solution, rather than come in with the answer and expect you to expedite it. Until you reach that point, you need to guide the patient to where he needs to be, even without him realising that's what you are doing. We will discuss this more deeply in Chapter 47.

CHAPTER 5

Let The Patient Do The Work

How long do doctors let patients talk before they interrupt them? Answers on the internet include 47 seconds, 27 seconds and even as low as 11 seconds. How accurate these figures are, whether they apply to all doctors, or all GPs, or only Australian GPs isn't what's important. What matters more is how long do **you** let a patient speak without interrupting?

There is a tension. A patient enters the room, and we use our opening line, carefully cultivated to avoid the "you're useless" comeback.

"How are you?" "Bloody awful of course, otherwise I wouldn't be here".

"What brings you in today?" "A car and then I walked".

"How can I help you?" "I can't be helped".

Which is why I prefer the phrase – "What can I do for you today?" or "What are we doing today?"

Registrars are often taught to get the agenda on the table. If you don't identify all the issues that the patient wants addressed you run the risk of going through a 20-minute consultation discussing mid-life screening, an intermittent headache and mild insomnia, only to have the patient mention on the way out that they've been getting chest pain for the past two weeks, worse over the past two days. Or after being fully examined for abdominal pain, redressing and sitting again, they mention that they'd like their back and leg moles checked.

So a common teaching is that you should encourage the patient to present their list. Ask "What would you like to address today?" And then "Anything else?" And then "Anything else?" again. And then "Is that it?" If they didn't come in with a written list, you've now created one and this technique sets a clear maximal boundary of what is to be covered. (See also Chapter 52.)

I think there is a significant problem with that approach, though I strongly acknowledge its utility, particularly when you don't know a patient particularly well.

The serious shortcoming is that the patient may not yet be ready to reveal their real concerns when they sit down at your desk. The concept of "ticket of entry" is really important. This is the idea that patients will present with one (minor) problem because consciously or unconsciously they are testing out the doctor – can she be trusted? Is she knowledgeable? Will she be respectful or judgemental?

Hammering the patient to lay out the whole agenda might break through that barrier. But it might also drive that real reason underground. The patient may now feel, even if they trust the doctor, that they've blown their chance to really speak openly, even if within a few minutes of the consultation starting, that they would really like to.

For this reason, the very best thing you can do for a patient is to listen. Just listen. Let the patient speak. Don't interrupt. Ask your opening question and then stop for as long as possible. When the patient finishes, don't ask anything. Say "Go on". When they run out of things to say, ask "What else?" Say "Uh-huh". Nod. Keep eye contact. But don't put your focus, vision, thoughts into the consultation until you are quite sure that the patient has completely run out of things to say. And then ask, "And is there anything else?" one more time.

Reflect for a moment on the commonest complaint patients make about doctors. "She kept me waiting so long". (That the second commonest complaint is contradictory is something we will address in Chapter 7.) And what is the patient doing in the waiting room whilst sitting there, nervously or otherwise, waiting to be seen? They are rehearsing what they are going to say when the doctor does call them in.

This means the patient has a speech ready. It might be well rehearsed and articulate; it might be stuttering and incoherent. But it will be something the patient wants the chance to say – else why did they invest so much time in preparing their response to that opening question?

The patient wants to tell you their story.

The sooner you interrupt with questions, or the more often you ask questions, the more likely they will lose their train of thought, the little details they are able to provide, the clues that may suggest there is an underlying agenda, reason or issue.

Sometimes it is necessary to interrupt and clarify the narrative, even early on. I suggest you do that with an apology – an emphasis that you are trying to understand the story, not that you are seeking different information or wanting to direct the conversation flow down the path you are interested in.

Once a patient has "spilled their guts", they are far more receptive to you then taking the lead, directing, drilling down. Let the patient speak. They will not listen until they've had their say.

CHAPTER 6

Hands And Heads

There are many reasons as a doctor to wash your hands. How many can you think of?

In essence, I think there are three. First – because of hygiene. Patients are filthy, germ riddled creatures with virus-teeming body-fluids on the inside and infectious organisms crawling all over the outside. Washing your hands whenever you touch a patient protects you from those risks. Of course, you could wear gloves whenever you touch a patient, but apart from the financial and environmental cost, there is a significant diagnostic, therapeutic and human benefit to touching skin with skin.

Washing hands immediately after touching a patient also prevents you becoming the fomite that spreads disease all through your consulting room. Think about all the surfaces you touch after examining a patient – the chair, your pen, the keyboard and mouse, the phone, the door handle ... Wash your hands after touching the patient, and all these surfaces are protected, even if not sterile.

The second reason to wash hands regularly, but particularly after examining a patient, is that it means that he sees you wash your hands. The assumption by the patient then is "She washed her hands after touching me – I can therefore feel comfortable that she washed her hands after touching the previous patient, and I have no need to fear something has just been transmitted."

(A brief digression. I note that correct hand-hygiene technique is to wash or use alcohol rub both before and after touching a patient. We also know how often doctors fail in this regard. I don't condone that but acknowledge the reality that washing before examination takes time, often results in wet hands examining a patient to everyone's discomfort, and sometimes results in the GP developing dermatitis. It is absolutely correct to wash before and after. But if, as most GPs tend to do, you only wash once, then I strongly suggest after.

I also recently observed my registrar use alcohol rub before examining a 2-year-old with lesions under his nose. I pointed out afterwards that the subsequent examination resulted in both the smell of alcohol putting the patient off, and ran the risk of touching alcohol-infused hands directly onto open wounds – which will certainly affect the doctor-patient relationship!)

But ultimately, I think the third reason is the most important:

Wash your hands after every examination - it gives you time to think.

In the simplest model, a consultation has three distinct phases. The first, the history, belongs to the patient. Though we may ask questions, the patient drives the agenda, provides the key information and has, so to speak, the power over what is happening.

The second phase, the examination, belongs to the doctor. The patient is essentially a passive participant in the process. We poke, prod, ask if something hurts, get them to roll to the left or bend to the right. But we are the directors of the show at that stage.

The third phase, the management phase, is a shared experience. Of course, the patient is expecting us to speak first, for we need to summarise what we've heard, seen, felt and found, explain our thoughts, provide a conclusion or diagnosis and then offer a plan. But after that it will be a shared experience of proposal, exploration of options and preferences and finally a commitment to act.

The opening moments of that third phase are therefore critical. Sometimes we know exactly what needs to happen, but we don't know how we will convince the patient. Other times we aren't sure what the diagnosis is and need to formulate a plan in the absence of the certainty that the patient has come in asking for. At other times we might need to break bad news the patient didn't expect or provide reassurance that the patient may not expect or want. (For example, a diagnosis of viral infection that does not need antibiotics may be precisely what the patient does not wish to hear.)

So those first moments of the third phase really matter. In some ways, they are the crux of bedside manner (a curious phrase, because in general practice the bedside is only where the examination phase takes place, not the history or management phase!) Getting your thoughts in order really matters.

Registrars however haven't always got a spiel for every situation. Whether encountering a particular condition for the first time, or a particular patient personality type for the first time, you will need to work out your phrasing before you start to speak.

One of the most embarrassing things that can happen to a doctor is to start an explanation, and then stumble over your words, the order of presentation, the analogy you use or to start and then backtrack and start again.

Even more embarrassing is to sit down in the doctor's chair, stare at the patient (or blankly at your computer screen) while the patient is staring at you, waiting for you to start speaking. And waiting. And waiting.

But if instead of going from the bed to your chair, you detour to the sink, turn on the tap, adjust the temperature, rinse your hands, pump some soap, wash your hands – thoroughly of course, carefully rubbing fingers and palms and even forearms – then rinsing off in the same deliberate manner, then drying them thoroughly, all before sitting down in your chair – you've just bought yourself an invaluable 30 seconds during which your movements have been slow and deliberate, but your thoughts have had an uninterrupted chance to sort themselves out.

In a particularly complex case, you might need to be extra careful about hand hygiene and wash them for sixty seconds. No-one will ever find this odd (unless it happens to be a mental health consultation!).

From the patient's perspective, you are just being a hygienic, careful doctor going through the motions that every TV show has taught them. And in my experience patients almost never talk or ask questions whilst you are washing your hands.

Yes, you can lengthen your thinking time by sitting down and immediately starting to type (perhaps muttering as I do "Give me a minute to write some notes – it helps me get my thoughts in order") but patients will sometimes feel free to interrupt at that point.

Washing your hands after every examination means you can now begin the third phase confident in your lead off that will carry you through to the end of the consultation.

CHAPTER 7

The Real Estate Principle

We've already noted in Chapter 5 that the number one complaint of patients is that they feel they have been kept waiting too long. What then is the number two complaint? "The doctor didn't spend enough time with me."

Research suggests that when judging the duration of a consultation without the aid of a clock, patients tend to underestimate the time spent, while doctors tend to overestimate. (The latter is an interesting phenomenon and may be related to our perceptions of the complexity of the consult and the busyness of our brain. We can think quickly, often in multiple layers and threads simultaneously, and whilst it would be nice if time-based remuneration counted each of those threads separately, it is the ticking of the clock that the Professional Services Review committee looks at!)

It's therefore important that a patient not just be *given* adequate time but to *feel* that she has been given that time. We need to "bulk up" the visit, so that she has a subconscious experience of a satisfying consultation.

Therefore:

Always put the patient on the couch.

You will recall we spoke of a consultation having three phases. Whilst commonly we continue to take some history during the examination phase, particularly in light of any findings the examination reveals, the drawback of doing that is that the patient is commonly so distracted by our questioning, she doesn't realise that we are checking her colour, hydration, skin colour or even pulse. I have even had patients deny an abdominal palpation took place because I've been so "successful" in distracting them during that examination!

By putting the patient on the couch whenever you examine her, you provide a memory jog that phase two – the examination – actually took place. I often have new patients complain that their previous doctor "didn't even examine me", and whilst that is probably true some of the time, when the same patient asks me to address the high blood pressure or murmur that the doctor told them about, it suggests that an examination did in fact take place – but the patient doesn't recall! Do what you can to avoid you being that doctor!

Breaking the consultation up into phases by putting the patient on the couch also provides her with a signal that the history phase is over and that now is the time for her to speak less and let you take charge. Of course, if there are important elements of history she only remembers now, we want her to speak, but hopefully we got all (or nearly all) of the story during the first phase.

Another motivation for creating the separation between history and examination that the couch provides is that if you are so inclined, it is perfectly acceptable for you to go silent during the examination phase. This may just provide a momentary respite from a day of conversation. It also gives you a chance to start synthesising your thoughts, at least about the history, and putting the examination into perspective. Silence means you can repeat "inspection, palpation, passive movement, active movement" to yourself, or remember the steps of a neuro exam, without having to process and respond to what the patient is saying.

On the other hand, if you don't mind talking during the examination, I observed a wonderful technique from my colleague Dr Peter Tribe. Peter is one of the kindest, gentlest doctors I've met, whose dog would sit under his desk while Peter played classical music in the consulting room.

Peter would often provide a running commentary as he examined the patient, which was foreign to me and struck me as quite odd, until I asked him to double check my findings on a patient. He did a cardiac auscultation and murmured to himself "good strong heart Mr Jones". And the look of pride in Mr Jones' eyes and the way he sat up with a smile a little straighter than before made me realise just how powerful that kind of exam-talk can be.

Let me deal with a couple of exceptions to this general rule. Many exams of course take place standing up rather than on the couch – examination of the spine and some other musculo-skeletal examinations, or examination of gait, balance and other neurology. But it would be rare indeed for the patient not to recognise those as an examination phase.

There is also a trend towards digital sphygmomanometers sitting on a doctor's desk rather than mercury machines hanging on the wall by the couch. It's certainly more convenient for the "just here for my blood pressure pills doc" visit, but it has many drawbacks. My observation is that GPs examine pulses much less often when using automated sphygmomanometers, and therefore are likely to miss picking up ectopics or atrial fibrillation. There is also much less likelihood of doing some incidental examination that happens almost automatically when you put a patient on the couch. The latter brings you physically closer to the patient and puts you essentially at eye-to-eye level. You'll notice jaundice, pallor, dehydration as well as neoplastic skin lesions close up that you simply won't find at desk distance.

You'll also protect your back more if you examine at proper height rather than try and bend over to look in an ear or check a mole. That might not matter to you early in your career but trust me, your back will eventually prefer a couch height exam!

The other big exception to the couch rule is infants. Here the technique is to always start examining the child on the parent's lap and in good position first time. If the parent isn't holding the child correctly and they wriggle, squirm or move, chances are they will either find the exam uncomfortable or something will hurt – eg that auroscope in their ear. The chances of having a hassle-free exam have now plummeted, even if you do get them held properly second time round.

I therefore always check that the parents are holding properly or give them clear instructions as to what I want. Ensure they are gently but firmly restraining the child before you get close – that way the child blames the parents for restricting their escape, not you!

One final reason for examining the patient on the couch ties in with our previous chapter. The patient having to move back to the chair (even if they haven't had to disrobe) gives you a few extra seconds to think about what you are going to say when you enter the third stage, the management phase of the visit.

Position, position, position is the key mantra of real estate. Turns out it also applies to general practice consultations.

CHAPTER 8

Fries With That

How do you know you are doing a good job? It's one of the hardest things to accurately judge. The Dunning-Kruger effect tells us that we are least likely to think we are doing a bad job, when we actually are!

Indeed, it is a curious paradox that the doctors who are the least skilled are often those most confident in their own abilities (and most critical of their colleagues), whilst those who are the best are the ones most plagued by self-doubt. By definition, half of all doctors are below median in their quality – yet few would think that of themselves.

How then can we judge ourselves objectively?

One option might be to look at your appointment book. If it's always full, that suggests patients aren't turning away from you. You must be meeting their needs, or at least their wants, if they keep coming back.

You could of course dig deeper. Are you full because of the general shortage of GPs? A particular shortage in your area? Are they coming because you are better than your colleagues – or because you are cheaper?

(I certainly don't believe that bulkbilling doctors are *ipso facto* worse than those who privately bill, but we can say that in general if a patient has the choice between two services otherwise equal, they will probably prefer the less expensive one. And some people by choice or necessity will trade off perception of quality of service for the certainty of savings.)

You might look at how many new patients you get, as a marker of your word-of-mouth reputation. Of course that is also going to be subject to factors like how many other doctors in the area have closed their books or taken leave. And if you have space in your appointment book for lots of new patients ... just maybe that means that the patients you have already seen may not be coming back to see you as much as you might have hoped. Perhaps they have gone elsewhere because you aren't actually meeting their wants ... or needs.

Patients are probably not the best judge of good doctors anyway. Patients are great judges of bedside manner – in fact, they are the only judges that matter. But they aren't great judges of clinical skills. A terrible doctor may be highly affable; a brilliant diagnostician may have poor social skills. It takes a long time for most patients to sort out the difference.

How else can we judge our quality? You might assess yourself against other criteria – perhaps an assessment of whether you are meeting the patient's agenda. If the patient walked in complaining of a rash, and you diagnose and treat her rash – you can go home satisfied. If at the end of the day you reflect back that you've done that with all the patients you met that day, you may be well satisfied. And your patients may well be satisfied as well.

But I will argue that this is still not the best guide to quality of care. Patients only know what they know. They only ask about that which is bothering them. If you address those issues – and only those issues – then you are addressing the patient's agenda for the consultation (which is highly appropriate!) – but abrogating your responsibility to have an agenda yourself.

At every consultation, a good GP does one thing the patient didn't ask for.

Your responsibility is to always dig deeper. That might be to unpeel the layers of the presenting problem.

Consider this consultation: "Janine – that rash is eczema. Try not to scratch, and here is some steroid cream. Read this handout on the causes and treatments. See me in a week if it's no better. Anything else? No? OK – see you later!"

Now compare that to this consult: "Janine ... we've worked out that rash is eczema, and we've worked out that it may well be coming from you scratching. Yet you don't catch yourself scratching very often. Are you scratching at night? Is your sleep disturbed? What's bothering you? Your sister has breast cancer? I'm so sorry. How are you coping with that? Let's check when your last mammogram was and take a more detailed family history to see if you need to go to a genetics clinic. Meanwhile we'll treat the eczema like this ..."

We will explore this in more detail in Chapter 31. In the meantime, here are other ways to dig deeper in a consultation.

One of the key differences between general practice and hospital medicine is continuity of care. Specialists treat illnesses. GPs treat people. We deal with acute illness, chronic illness and preventative health. We treat individuals, but we also treat families and communities.

So for every patient there is an ongoing cycle of care. When did you last check Janine's blood pressure? Easy! What about her weight? Less common. Her waist/hip ratio? Nearly never! When do you think about her immunisation status? What will trigger you to arrange a home medication review? Are her conditions complex enough for her to warrant a care plan? Do you know if her rheumatologist and her physiotherapist are each writing to the other to inform what is going on? Or are they relying on you to keep everyone in the loop? If you ever wrote an indefinite referral, have you updated that specialist with Janine's new antihypertensive, and maybe the adverse reaction (but not allergy) that she had to amlodipine? When was her last skin check? FOBT? Mammogram? Chlamydia screen? How is her mental health – not depressed, but we know that her son is a troubled teen ... how is he going and how is she coping? Have you asked? When is her next holiday – and where will she be travelling and does she need immunisations or an antiemetic for the trip?

Even things we did really well need to be done again. You took a thorough history when Janine joined your practice 14 years ago? Great! When was the last time you checked, updated (and recorded the date of updating) her family and social history? Her new job (and new work phone number)? Her parents may not have had any major illnesses back then ... but developed diabetes, heart disease and had a CVA in the intervening years!

You don't need to do all these things at every visit. You couldn't, even if you allowed 30 minutes for every consultation. But over a period of time – a cycle of care in the real meaning of the word – you need to think about these things thoroughly and act on them.

Yes, it is exhausting – both the cognitive load to always keep thinking about what else we can do to optimise every patient's health, and the time factors when our day is already packed, and any shorter than normal consultation is a blessing that allows us to claw back a minute or two, after we gifted an extra unbooked double-consultation's worth to the teenager who entered and burst out crying.

Nonetheless, if you can look back on your day, and honestly say you did one thing for each patient that they didn't ask for – then you can indeed know that you are doing a great job as a GP.

CHAPTER 9

Words And Numbers

We've already discussed – believe the patient. We've already discussed listen to the patient, and take a good history, and nothing replaces an examination, and that you should listen to your gut as much as you listen to the experts.

But we live in a modern world, with the availability of tests that our forebears could only imagine. Just in my career we've moved from x-ray, ultrasound and the beginnings of CT scans to low dose-HRCT, MRI, PET scans, nuclear medicine, bone densitometry, CACS and a whole host of imaging techniques at a cost and availability that was unfathomable. If you want to know how much radiology has evolved, please look up images of pneumoencephalography and compare that to a suburban MRI.

Similarly, though our "basic bloods" (what a thoughtless term!) haven't changed – FBE, UEs, LFTs, TSH, BSL, and then whatever else you want to add on – the number of exotic, sophisticated tests expands monthly. That oncologists come up with tests I don't know doesn't surprise me – I made a decision as an intern that oncology was something that changed so rapidly and was so critical that I wouldn't ever dabble in trying to keep up. But now rheumatologists keep finding new antibodies every month. Genomics wasn't even a word when I began general practice.

It's completely normal to want to use tests – old or new – to diagnose and therefore treat our patients, but there are two fundamental problems.

First – tests miss things. No matter how sophisticated the test, no test is perfect. And yes, newer tests are less imperfect – but to believe a test is, by definition, to not believe the patient. If you could rely entirely on the patient, you wouldn't need to do the test. But if you rely entirely on the test, you are saying that you don't need any input from the patient. Clearly, we need both.

Tests also miss things because of the inherent inaccuracy of pathology operators – human or machine. We love numbers so we don't think about their imprecision. Whether a sodium is 144 (normal) or 146 (abnormal) makes absolutely no difference. If you construe that degree of variation as significant, you have no business being a GP!

But when it comes in particular to radiology, we aren't dealing with numbers but with interpretation. No matter how sophisticated the machine, the eyes and brains of the radiologist matter the most. And her style of writing reports also matters the most. Finally, how accessible she is to phone calls – including after hours - matters the most.

Whilst radiologists advertise themselves on the quality of their equipment ("we have the latest 2^n scanner"), what really matters is the quality of the radiologist. Pathology is (if you will forgive the sexist alliteration) 90% the machine, 10% the man. But radiology is 90% the man, 10% the machine. (See also Chapter 40.)

What is true of radiology is also true of histology – even with the move to standardised reporting, you will eventually learn the nuance and style of your preferred pathologists, and when exactly you need to express doubts about what you are reading.

The second problem is that tests find things – things that do not matter. The exact percentage may be the subject of debate, but it's useful to quote to patients seeking weakly indicated imaging, that 50% of brain MRIs find a lesion NOT in the region of the brain where there was concern. Well now what? Are you just going to ignore a lesion in the brain? Or are you going to biopsy an incidental finding that's causing no symptoms at all, has probably been there for a long period of time, and is almost certainly not clinically concerning? Or are you going to spend the next three to six months worrying about whether there is a lesion there that matters and then repeat the MRI a couple of times "just to be sure"?

No – it's very, very often better not to order a test of dubious value than it is to do a test just to check things out. There is a well-established adage – before you do a test, ask yourself, what will you do if the test is positive? What will you do if the test is negative? If the answer is the same, don't do the test.

Mathematically there is a well-established principle that calculates the utility of a test, called Bayes Theorem. In essence, this states that how likely a test result is actually correct - not a false positive or negative - depends on how likely it was to get that result before you did the test.

To take an extreme example - if an hCG test comes back positive in a chromosomally male patient, it is not an indicator that he is pregnant! The pretest probability of that was zero, and the post-test likelihood is that this is a false positive, at least as far as pregnancy goes. (He could of course, have a germ cell tumour - but presumably that was a possibility you considered when ordering the test.)

When you read Chapter 14 in this light - almost every pathology test has a 5% false positive rate. If the chance that the patient has a particular condition is less than 5% to begin with, then a positive result is more likely to be false than true!

That doesn't mean you shouldn't ever order low likelihood tests. There are unlikely but high risk conditions that warrant low-yield tests. But do so with open eyes, open mind and an understanding that the test results are not necessarily of significance.

The power of pathology and radiology is immense. But always remember that

Investigations are merely a numeric or pictorial approximation of the patient's clinical condition.

If a test result doesn't fit the clinical picture - if something isn't there that should be, or is there that shouldn't be, think again.

And if it still doesn't make sense, then remember that radiologists and pathologists are consultants - so consult! You should probably be calling your pathologists and radiologists at least weekly, if not daily. Which test should I order? What does this result mean? How can I be sure and how sure need I be? In most cases, they will be delighted to look up from their microscope or away from their computer screen to discuss the human to whom the pictures and numbers belong.

CHAPTER 10

We Are All Ducklings

When I was in Grade 4, a student-teacher involved me in a research study on how many repetitions it takes children to learn – and two weeks later, re-learn – a list of eight nonsense words. Here they are: zil, nam, jox, foz, gek, pab, wug and kiv.

Why do I remember these gibberish words from over 50 years ago so vividly? Because

What we learned when we were young stays imprinted – rightly or wrongly.

The early learning we do is not just an additional piece in a jigsaw puzzle – it becomes the very scaffolding on which all other learning takes place. Early learning is the framework that everything subsequent is either compared to or contrasted with.

It's awfully hard to switch from a drug class you've successfully prescribed for 20 years to another, newer class even if the novel agents promise better efficacy or fewer side-effects. (And let's set aside for a moment the fact that our knowledge of the side-effect profile of most new drug classes doesn't show up for five to ten years.)

At the start of your general practice career you will both admire the experience of your supervisors and be a little taken aback at how entrenched they are in some quaint or antiquated medical habits. You will pledge to always remain up-to-date. And if you practice long enough, the registrars you teach will secretly feel the same about you.

Learning medicine is hard. But forgetting things (abandoning them, not being unable to recall!) is even harder.

Yet unlearning no-longer-true truths is as important as gathering new knowledge.

It isn't only knowledge that is imprinted early on in our careers. Even more so – it is values and attitude.

I have repeatedly told my teenagers that the most important question to ask when interviewing for their first job is what teaching will they get. Not the pay, not the hours, not the benefits, not the prospects of internal growth or promotion or becoming a partner. Just – who will teach me? What will they teach me? How will they teach me?

What I particularly want is them to learn a work ethic, what it means to put in a solid effort, what it means to care for patient or client. If they become GPs, I want them to appreciate the difference between performing consultations and providing care for patients.

As superficial as it is, first impressions count. Without a context or background information, we tend to accept as true all that we hear from those more expert, experienced or knowledgeable than us. But how do we know they are more expert, experienced or knowledgeable until we have some perspective from which to draw on and judge what our mentors and teachers are saying? Why are you believing anything I am saying in this book?!

Indeed, ask yourself - Why do practices teach registrars? And in particular, why take on T1 registrars (those in their first term of general practice)? They know nothing about general practice. They ask questions all the time. They interrupt the supervisor, they make mistakes of ignorance, they bill incorrectly, they haven't learned how to handle illness and they certainly haven't learned how to handle patients. They are entitled to far more teaching time and can have far less demands placed on them for patient load. Despite popular perception amongst registrars, they are financially the least worthwhile registrars for practices to take on.

Why would any practice in its right mind take on early term registrars?

Because those who love T1s know that this is the best time to really shape not just the medicine, but the values of a future general practitioner.

I urge you to choose your first general practice terms very, very carefully. Don't focus on pay, don't focus on rosters. Ask how much formal one-on-one teaching you will get, and more importantly, how much informal, over a cup of coffee conversation you will get. How often do doctors drop in on each other? How often do doctors call each other in – not just registrars, but all the GPs? Who will tell you "war stories"? Who will you chat to over lunch?

Ask about the rosters and nursing home visits and the on-call, not to avoid them but to experience them! Even if you decide you'll never do another home visit in your life afterwards, until you've tried it out, you will have no idea of just how valuable they can be – for you, as well as the patient.

Although my view is unpopular, this is why I feel so strongly that registrars should not do twelve months in the same practice, and particularly not in their first year. Yes, continuity of care is the hallmark of general practice and in twelve months you will experience much more of that than in six months. However, you have your entire professional lifetime where that happens.

But if you spend twelve months in your very first practice, then that clinic's values alone will become the prism through which you will see every practice and consultation for the rest of your life. And it's important that you develop that through multiple, diverse perspectives.

CHAPTER 11

Spending Time

If there is limited time in a consultation to do a history and examination and management plan, how then do you best allocate that time? This is often a question of candidates for the RACGP or ACRRM exam, but it is more important to ask that question when planning your consultation.

There is an adage that in general practice 70% of the time you make the diagnosis from the history, 20% of the time from the physical examination and only 10% of the time from investigations and tests.

It therefore seems reasonable to allocate significantly more time to the history than any other aspect of the consultation. Note that these figures refer to the diagnostic process, and don't include time to be spent in explaining your diagnosis or providing a management plan. So don't interpret it to mean that 70% of your whole appointment slot should be history alone.

Nonetheless, the corollary of this 70/20/10 division should be pretty clear. If you don't know what's wrong by the time you put the patient on the bed, you are in trouble!

In my early days of general practice, around thirty years ago, a young woman saw me because she was suffering from orange vision. Everything had an orange shade. This rang vague bells – digoxin toxicity can cause yellow or orange vision and so I grilled her multiple times about whether she was taking digoxin. Whether anyone in her family was taking it and she was accidentally ingesting it. I gently probed if anyone might be slipping her tablets in an effort to harm her. I wondered if she was suffering Munchausen's syndrome. Nothing.

I asked every question I could think of regarding physical health, psychological disease and emotional stress – but everything came up blank. And physical examination – with no idea what to look for – showed normal vision, normal eyes and no icterus.

We should have moved on to investigation – but what tests would I even order? And so, fortuitously, I went back to history.

I probed exercise, sleep and diet, and then in desperation and for no particular reason asked if she drank much tea or coffee.

"Oh – I like coffee", she said. "How many do you drink?" I asked.

"We have one of those new coffee machines in the office and I make a few", she answered rather casually.

Had I been asking about alcohol, I would have been suspicious of the vague response but here I really expected a socially normal answer. Nonetheless, I asked one more question.

"How many?"

"Oh – about 20 a day."

I leapt out of my chair and for one of the very few times in my career reached for a pharmacology textbook. Sure enough, yellow vision is a recognised symptom of caffeine intoxication.

Lesson learned. I now routinely ask every new patient, and any patient with unusual symptoms how many caffeinated drinks they take. But more importantly, I learned the lesson that

If the history is unrevealing take more history.

Most of the time – certainly not always – you should have a pretty good idea of what you are going to find when you examine the patient before you actually start. Of course you must go in with an unbiased mind and open eyes and ears. You won't find things you weren't expecting if you make assumptions about what will be revealed.

Similarly, there are some things that simply won't show up in a history. And others that aren't identifiable without tests. But in the vast majority of cases, examination and investigation confirm what we suspect rather than shock us with something unexpected.

As with so many other things in general practice, it's a matter of balance. At some point, extra history becomes a case of diminishing returns. There's no clear formula for when it's time to move from history to exam, other than when you've run out of useful questions to ask.

But when you reach that point of frustration, (see Chapter 28) try and squeeze out one or two more questions – even something completely out of left field. You never know what you might learn.

CHAPTER 12

Say Something

Having listed some of our patients' most common complaints, I'd like to list one of mine: there is an expectation of perfection of health care that does not seem to exist in other industries. Indeed, if we made the sorts of mistakes that I have frequently seen made by solicitors, accountants, town planners, traffic engineers and especially bank valuers, people would die.

Curiously, our own patients don't expect perfection from us as much as they do from the profession as a whole. I think this reflects the interesting experience that if you ask the populace how much they trust and respect various professions, doctors rank highly but often not in the first two or three. When asked how much they trust and respect THEIR doctor, GPs rank way above any other profession.

In other words, our relationship with patients tends to be stronger than their faith in the profession as a whole. As a result, patients do not resent us if we aren't perfect. They (by and large) understand that diagnoses take time and involve a process; that sometimes we need a second opinion; that we can't perform every operation ourselves and that sometimes there is indeed nothing that can be done for their condition.

But a patient still wants to feel that they have received value in the consultation. Every visit to the doctor is expensive – whether that is financial, or through the time and effort of booking, arriving, waiting (and waiting and waiting!) and above all the stress of the consultation itself. Denial is a powerful tool and if patients are to abandon that to come and see us, it behoves us to make it worth their while.

What then do we do if we are caught in diagnostic uncertainty? The patient has come with symptoms, but more importantly come with concern about their symptoms. You aren't providing an answer? Then what was the point of the patient coming?

But there is something you can do for this patient.

If you don't know what it is, tell the patient what it's not.

Patients often imagine the worst. They very often fear it. Every mole might be a melanoma, a nodule must be a cancer. Forgetting a word must mean dementia. Not every patient feels this way – but enough do.

In classic teaching, you are meant to specifically ask about the patients' ICE – ideas, concerns and expectations.

You job is to allay their fear. Remember Chapter 1 – You have to deal with the patient's agenda before you deal with your own. Until you have dealt with their concerns ("Am I going to walk out of here with a death sentence?") they won't listen to or absorb the wonderful management plan and explanation that you provide. Even more so if you say I have no idea what this is, but some path lab, radiologist or surgeon might.

But if you can commence your commentary with the reassurance that "Whatever it is, I am confident this isn't a melanoma" (or dementia or a heart attack), you will engage the patient in the rest of the consultation and illness episode because you have managed to delve beyond their words and into their thoughts. They will be profoundly grateful!

CHAPTER 13

Say Something (Again!)

I had the pleasure of being an examiner for the RACGP exams for many years, acting the part of a patient. Depending on the case instructions, most stations gave the candidates 3 minutes to read the background information – which might have just been a patient summary or might be what the presenting problem had been at an imagined previous consultation and providing test results that needed to be interpreted and presented to the patient.

Candidates were usually seen by two experienced GP examiners – one who role-played and the other who was the observer. One particular case comes to mind. I presented to a patient with change in bowel habit, and the registrar candidate did, I thought, a good job of taking a history, evaluating that a colonoscopy was called for and explaining to me that it was important that I book and attend the test because there was the possibility of cancer.

The examiners were expected to collaborate on the scoring, and I asked, out of courtesy, my co-examiner's thoughts about what to record for communication skills. My pen was already hovering to tick the "near perfect" box when, to my great surprise, the other examiner said "Fail".

I was shocked. He explained that one must never tell a patient that there was even the possibility of cancer. It was a devastating blow and could easily lead to a patient leaving the clinic, going home and committing suicide.

I generally have great respect for the elder statesmen of general practice, and I would normally have deferred to his opinion. But I felt in this case that this was as patronising an approach as one could possibly have.

Perhaps my view is skewed by working in a suburb and practice where health literacy is well above average. Most of my patients, and I suspect most of the populace, would at least have some suspicion that a change in bowel habit can be serious, and if something in the bowel is serious then cancer is a possibility.

They may not say it – but I believe they are thinking it. If one of our main responsibilities is to make sure the patient leaves the consulting room feeling better than when they came in, then it is up to us to address the issue that is worrying them most even if they don't mention it.

We need to peel back the layers of the consultation. You may have a very clear-eyed perspective on how unlikely a particular diagnosis is. But patients don't have the benefit of your training and experience. Many will fear the worst even if they can't put a name to it.

Patients are taught to fear any new lump. You might know it's a dermatofibroma or a lipoma or a sebaceous cyst. But no matter how clearly you say that this is not a problem, until you specifically say, "It isn't cancer", they will not relax.

The same applies to any symptom that sits in the public eye. Any skin lesion will be a melanoma until you reassure otherwise. Any shake of the hand might be Parkinson's. Any odd neuro symptom will raise the spectre of multiple sclerosis. And forgetting anything – a word, a birthday, an appointment – will lead inevitably to the fear of dementia.

And so you need to be very alert to the concerns that a patient raises. You need to listen to their words and you need to read their body language. You need to look at their face whilst examining their abdomen or knees for a flinch of discomfort that indicates pain they might not mention. And you need to be alert to all the things that a patient dares not name but are the real concern that they are coming to be reassured about.

So, no matter how remote the possibility, if there is any chance the patient (or their family) are thinking about serious diagnoses, you have to address the issue.

If the patient doesn't mention cancer, MS, Alzheimer's, Parkinson's (or MND) – you must.

I choose these diseases because I think they are the commonest fear generators. They are common enough that patients have heard of them, and nasty enough that patients are terrified of them. MND is in brackets because it is much rarer, and only the more health literate patients will know it.

You are welcome to add to this list. I would not want you to paradoxically trigger panic in your patients by refuting more and more obscure diseases, but it does pay to keep an eye on the popular press to anticipate the questions that people will ask. Perhaps more importantly, the questions that people won't ask but will be wondering.

Thus, if there is a story in the tabloid media about Buruli ulcers or Zika virus or an epidemic of kidney stones, it pays to actively acknowledge that when a patient presents with "illness-adjacent" symptoms.

One related concept. Whenever a patient comes in "just for a checkup", you should always ask what led to this. The "Angelina Jolie effect" and the "Shane Warne phenomenon" brought lots of patients in for health checkups who specifically wanted breast cancer excluded or heart disease ruled out, even without any symptoms at all. Often as not, they were sent in by their spouses rather than deciding to come in for themselves.

If you don't think about what triggered the visit, you won't identify what the patient is too scared to ask for - and you haven't helped them with their greatest need. We will discuss this much more deeply in Chapter 31.

(And for those who are wondering what happened to the candidate, we eventually agreed to disagree and wrote "split vote" on the exam marking form. I was subsequently told it would be ignored, and his communication skills mark would be based on his performance at other stations.)

CHAPTER 14

Do The Maths

I am surprised how many registrars can't give an answer to the question – what do we mean when we say a test is abnormal?

Of course it means that the result is outside the normal range. But that just dodges the question. What is the normal range? And how did we work it out?

For most tests – and it's important that you understand which ones this does and doesn't apply to – the normal range is calculated by taking lots of samples of apparently normal, healthy people and plotting the result on a normal distribution ("bell curve"). We then define normal to be plus or minus two standard deviations from the mean of that range.

So – do you remember what proportion of people lie inside that ±2SD range? If you do – congratulations! In my experience you lie outside the normal range if you know how many lie inside the normal range!

The answer, in case you've forgotten your high school statistics, is about 95%. In round terms, ±1SD, covers about two-thirds of the population; ±2SD covers about 95% and ±3SD includes 99.7% of the population.

Now remember, this represents a normal, healthy population. So by definition, 5% of healthy, normal people are outside the normal distribution. True, usually it's only by a very small amount. But that is also important. It means that many, if not most, minor abnormalities are probably not significant. They are probably just the result of a minor statistical outlier – perhaps re-read Chapter 9.

Let's get a little mathematical. If a healthy person has a 95% chance that a test is normal and 5% that it will be abnormal, how often will a patient who undergoes two blood tests have both tests come back normal versus at least one of them being abnormal?

Well, 95% of people will be normal on the first test. And 95% of those will be normal on the second test. So 95% of 95% is

90.25%. Nearly 10% of patients will have an abnormality if you order two tests, even if they are completely healthy.

Let's extend that out:

Number of tests	Chance all are normal	Number of tests	Chance all are normal	Number of tests	Chance all are normal
1	95.0%	6	73.5%	11	56.9%
2	90.3%	7	69.8%	12	54.0%
3	85.7%	8	66.3%	13	51.3%
4	81.5%	9	63.0%	14	48.8%
5	77.4%	10	59.9%	15	46.3%

Each line is 95% of the line above.

Notice that once you order 14 tests, you are more likely to get at least one abnormal result than for all the results to come back normal! Hence, the likelihood

Fourteen tests equals an abnormality.

Well, I hear you cry, that's not going to happen! I never order 14 tests on a single patient!

Actually, you do – every day. When you order electrolytes, liver function and a blood count, you are ordering (depending on your lab) 30 different tests: sodium, potassium, chloride, bicarbonate, urea, creatinine, eGFR, AST, ALT, GGT, ALP, bilirubin, total protein, albumin, globulin, haemoglobin, white cell count, platelets, neutrophils, lymphocytes, monocytes, eosinophils, basophils, red cell count, haematocrit, mean corpuscular volume, mean corpuscular haemoglobin, mean corpuscular haemoglobin concentration, red cell distribution width and maybe a reticulocyte count.

OK – I confess, I cheated. Obviously total protein, albumin and globulin are two tests, not three. Clearly all the red cell indices are tightly bound together as different views of what is essentially the same test. And even sodium, potassium and chloride aren't independent tests as the "95% of 95%" calculation requires.

Nonetheless, it is easy to see that ordering fourteen tests on a single pathology request is very easy to achieve, and with that, the likelihood of an abnormality.

As unappealing as it might be if you don't love probability, you need to review Bayes theorem. Understand about pre- and post-test probability; positive and negative predictive values; sensitivity and specificity; false positives and false negatives. You should not order a test unless you know what to do with the result, which means knowing whether the result is reliable and believable.

And, having found one, what to do about a minor abnormality is sometimes very difficult. You might chase it and chase it to no avail. Or you might find something at its earliest stages because you were so diligent. The trade off between over-investigation and under-diagnosis is one you will deal with every day. Be aware that there is no right answer as to how many tests are the right number to order. It isn't something to be determined by an econocrat – though perhaps they can decide who pays for the tests. The utility of a test is a function of your discussion with the patient as to the likelihood of abnormality, the seriousness of what you are looking for, the patient's degree of concern and your tolerance of risk. (See also Chapter 29.)

I'd like also to briefly comment on the difference between normal and recommended ranges. Sodium sits in a tight range. Cholesterol is open ended. As a young doctor, my labs reported normal cholesterol as <6.5 mmol/l. This simply meant that 97.5% of results fell under that limit. Naturally, the lower tail of the bell curve was still considered normal, even though it fell outside the range.

But then we got more and more focussed on cholesterol as a risk factor and took to describing desirable cholesterol ranges rather than normal ones. Recommended levels were then reduced to 6.0 and later 5.5 and now 5.0 (and even lower!) Suddenly lots of previously normal people had abnormal results without their numbers changing!

This discussion has real-life implications. Diabetes diagnoses surged when the cut off was lowered from 7.8 mmol/l to 7.0. It was described as an epidemic of diabetes, but really it was a redefinition.

Similarly, labs often report normal Vitamin D levels as being greater than 50 nmol/l ... but recommended levels as over 70. In other words, a big chunk of the normal population hasn't reached recommended levels. Should most of the population be on supplementation for the next winter, year or lifetime? It all depends on what you mean by abnormality.

A final confession. When I quote my own rules to registrars, I mostly can't remember the order, so I just make up the numbers. Rule 24 could be just about anything depending on my mood for the day. But rule 14 is always rule 14 for what should now be memorable reasons!

CHAPTER 15

Metamorphosis

How do you know when a mole is a melanoma? When do you worry enough to do something about it, particularly in a hurry? You can always wait 3 months and then review - but when would you feel that is a problem? In other words - when is a mole an emergency?

The classic answer is that a mole is a concern if it is changing - particularly size, shape, colour or is bleeding. But blood is a different hue to melanin, so I guess we can call that a change in colour, and whilst topologically a wedding ring and a car tyre are the same, the different size is enough to conceptually regard them as different shapes.

It occurred to me recently, when a registrar wanted a simple principle on when to send a patient to hospital, that what applies to moles applies to patients as a whole.

An emergency is when a patient changes shape or colour.

Cyanosis, jaundice, ash-grey pallor, haemorrhage each have active causes, some of which aren't immediately life threatening. But until we've worked them up, we don't know that they are not. An emergency may not always need referral to an ED, but it will always need urgent investigation and/or treatment.

Similarly, a bone pointing in the wrong direction, a missing digit or quinsy are all sufficient changes in shape to warrant immediate treatment in the practice or in hospital. In order to not miss heart attacks or strokes, I will stretch and say that the facial droop of a TIA or the grimace accompanying central chest pain can also be regarded as a change of shape.

I emphasise that this rule of thumb does not provide perfect sensitivity and specificity. Plenty of heart attacks present with subtle symptoms that need a high index of suspicion, not with textbook features. Still, this concept will adequately separate the majority of cases into their correct category of urgency.

There's one group that this doesn't apply to and who need a different rule, which is identifying a mental health emergency. For this I fall back on the first 15 minutes of my first day as a medical student in psychiatry rotation.

Our professor simply told us that we should talk to the patient for about an hour and then ask ourselves two questions. Could we understand why the patient felt the way they did? If the answer was yes, then (using the now outdated terminology) the patient was suffering a neurosis. If the answer was no, then the patient was suffering a psychosis.

The second question was to ask ourselves how we felt. That was the diagnostic category of the patient. If we felt angry – the patient had a form of paranoia; if we felt sad – the patient had depression; and if we felt totally confused – the patient had schizophrenia!

It's a very rough diagnostic model – some might call it Psychiatry for Dummies – but for non-specialists it's a very handy tool for working out how serious a patient's psychiatric presentation is. If a patient, overwhelmed by home, work and financial circumstances is suffering fleeting thoughts of suicide which they consider and scrap, that's probably a normal response. They are contemplating all their options and rejecting the ones that aren't productive. "How do I escape my unbearable life? I could quit my job and move to Samoa – but I won't. I could kill myself – but I don't want my family to suffer. I could pay a hitman to take out my manager and the Commissioner of Taxation – but then I'd probably rot in jail." They are all ideas that are worthy of consideration, momentarily, and if immediately discarded we can understand why the patient feels that way.

For some patients however, having those thoughts even fleetingly is frightening and unacceptable, even if they recognise how improper acting on them would be. Don't ignore the patient's distress about their feelings, but neither do you have to regard those thoughts as an emergency.

But when you can't understand why a patient's situation is so dire as to warrant the feelings they are expressing – particularly if their response is to actively plan suicide, which I suppose is the ultimate change in shape and colour – then you should certainly regard that as a psychiatric emergency worthy of immediate care.

Further study and experience will provide you with much greater knowledge of how to handle perceived, potential and real emergencies, both physical and psychological. Until then, I hope these rules of thumb are a helpful starter to thinking about what constitutes an emergency.

CHAPTER 16

Mother Knows Best

When my daughter was two years old, my wife Ruth turned to me and said "Yoni is pale, she's tired, she's grumpy. I think she needs to see a doctor." I patiently explained that two-year-olds don't spend hours in the sun and of course she was tired - she was spending her days running around playing.

She gave me a disapproving look, but nothing more. A few weeks later, she repeated "Yoni's pale and tired. She's grumpy. I want her to see a doctor!" This time it was I who gave her a disapproving look, but we dutifully went to see our family GP (everybody needs a GP!), an experienced and very patient doctor who appropriately took a history, conducted an exam and explained that two year-olds typically have only two speeds, on and off, so her tiredness was a normal healthy behaviour. Ruth seemed less than convinced.

A month or two later she said "Yoni's pale. She's tired. She's grumpy. I want to see a paediatrician." Despite my strong feeling that this was a waste of time and resources, it was clear that years of telling my wife that GPs can handle almost anything hadn't penetrated. A specialist appointment was duly arranged.

Our paediatrician, kind and gentle, teased out the history, explored diet and sleep patterns and behavioural issues. He did a thorough exam. His verdict? She's a normal, healthy two-year-old. Ruth's lip almost bled, she was biting so hard.

A few months went by. Yoni was happily skipping on the beach. Ruth turned to me and said: "Yoni is pale. She's tired. She's grumpy." I pointed out that she had seen me, an excellent GP, and a great paediatrician. We all had told her that there was nothing wrong.

"I don't care. I want a blood test", said Ruth. At this I drew the line. It was one thing to take Yoni from doctor to doctor, quite another to subject her to unnecessary needles and pain. However my objections were met with the sort of withering look that makes fathers quake and husbands quiver. Our GP arranged a blood test.

Yoni's ferritin was 2.

It's a well-known mantra, but it can't be emphasised often enough.

Always believe the patient – especially the mother.

Patients don't always know what is wrong. But they very often know that something is wrong. And even if their conclusions are wrong, their primary instinct that something isn't right, is by definition correct.

Why always correct? Because patients don't suffer diseases, they suffer dis-eases. When a patient comes in they aren't saying "I have diagnosis X". They are saying "I don't feel like I think I should." Which you should always believe! You have no basis not to!

It may be that the patient's dis-ease is physical, it may be emotional or it may be a physical manifestation of an emotional, mental or psychiatric issue. But the dis-ease is real enough.

Parents are particularly attuned to detecting minor changes in their children. They may misinterpret the symptoms or the signs; they may be wrong in their diagnosis. But the initial trigger of their concern is very real and your role is to identify not the disease, but the cause of the patient's or parent's dis-ease.

CHAPTER 17

Buyers Are Liars

Patients are really bad at medicine. Which is good, otherwise we'd be out of a job!

So when a patient comes in waving a newspaper article they've cut out, or worse, a Dr Google article they've printed off, we clearly don't start with the assumption that they are right. We go back to basics – ask them for the story from the beginning, examine, investigate.

Commonly, patients will present complaining of their migraine. But explore further and it will turn out that they are a 50-year-old who has never had a migraine before. The headache is band-like or was thunderclap; they have huge stress or uncontrolled BP.

A patient says they are depressed. In reality they have anxiety. They come in saying they have bleeding from haemorrhoids. A great way for you to miss a bowel cancer. They claim to have a hernia. You can easily overlook their inguinal lymph nodes.

Listen carefully to everything a patient says – but don't believe a word of it. You aren't doing them a disservice – you are doing exactly what your role is.

Similarly when a patient describes how poor another doctor is, be very cautious in accepting that at face value. We recently had a patient who switched from seeing me to another GP within our clinic. When he was asked why, he explained "I've got a pain in me armpit. It's a lump. The other doctor (me), he looked at it 20 years ago. Could be cancer. Hasn't checked it since."

Actually, I had reviewed his lump semi-regularly, and because he had expressed concern, had arranged an ultrasound (all clear) less than four months previously! Had he gone to another practice instead of my colleague, I would never have known and in that doctor's mind my reputation would be permanently stained. Don't you be the one guilty of dismissing another doctor unless you are in possession of all the facts.

So when a patient complains of a migraine ask them, "Can you describe the pain without using the word migraine?" If they complain of tiredness, ask them to distinguish between fatigue, sleepiness and lack of energy. When they use the word dizziness, ask them to describe whether they mean unsteadiness, vertigo or feeling faint.

Even words that seem to defy misunderstanding can be misused by patients. I can't count the number of times patients have confused the terms constipation and diarrhoea, and even if used correctly, constipation could mean hard stool, infrequent stool or straining at stool.

What is true of all patients is particularly true of parents. Their exhaustion or their anxiety often leads them to wrong conclusions in their (highly appropriate) urgent need to understand what is happening with their children. Parents might insist their infant's crying is pathological when it's just three-month colic. They will insist their child has ADHD when really they are just showing normal two-year old behaviours.

Parents gather health information from multiple sources, not all reliable. Play-groups are a fantastic resource and support network but we aren't privy to the power dynamics and voices in the crowd that can lead to group-think. The internet is reliably unreliable and social media even worse. Patients, but particularly parents, need answers and can gravitate to whichever ones are offered confidently, regardless of origin or accuracy.

At the same time, they can be in complete denial of genuine problems. Many a parent will refuse to accept that their child has an intellectual disability, an eating disorder or is morbidly overweight. The latter is often taken, no matter how phrased, as an attack on the parent rather than a concern for the child.

Parents can even refute the evidence in front of their eyes if they feel it reflects on their care. I recall one teenager who came in with a sore scapula after doing a somersault in her Physical Education class. Examination revealed the worst scoliosis I've seen. It had clearly been there and evolving for years – but her mother had never noticed and completely denied that there was any asymmetry and if there was, it could only be a few days old.

It's therefore incumbent upon us to

Believe nothing the patient tells you.

Rely on your own history and observations, your own diagnoses and conclusions.

How do we reconcile the need to believe everything the patient tells us and believing nothing? First by understanding the difference between believing the patient who says something is wrong and being cautious about the patient telling us what is wrong. Symptoms belong to the patient, diagnosis belongs to the doctor. We will discuss this again in Chapter 30.

Second, practice thinking simultaneously on different levels – get subjectively and empathically inside the mind of the patient – why are they feeling this way – whilst at the same time work through your objective process of assessment.

Nobody promised you general practice was easy!

CHAPTER 18

It's Hard To Hit A Moving Target

We chose to be doctors not vets! We like to talk to patients and we want to find out about their lives. We want to hear their stories – both medical and social. And we love that they can walk in and tell us what is bothering them.

So why the hell do we have to deal with paediatrics? The younger the patient, the more veterinarian-like is the consultation. We may get minimal or no history, we may get unreliable physical findings, and we may have a barely or even totally uncooperative patient who wishes only to get out of the room as fast as possible.

On the other hand, these are the very patients who need most careful assessment. A child can go from well to unwell to sick to flat to dead in almost the blink of an eye, and we need to identify that as early as possible and treat hard and fast! We certainly don't want to over-investigate a child with painful blood tests and uncomfortable x-rays – that's a guarantee for long-term doctor-aversion. Neither child, parent nor emergency department will appreciate referrals for symptoms that turn out to be minor viruses.

But even more, we do not want to miss something that matters. As my paediatric registrar Dr Richard McNeill taught – "No one says thank-you for a dead baby." An unnecessary lumbar puncture is profoundly unpleasant. A necessary lumbar puncture not done is a disaster.

How then to distinguish between the child that is merely miserable and the child who is imminently septic? There are a few useful clinical rules of thumb.

Learn to assess hydration in a child. Babies really need to do only four things - drink, wee, poo and sleep. If they are doing those well, they will probably be ok till the next time you see them.

The other big factor is simply how unwell the child looks. A fever on its own is not a major issue if the child is otherwise well. That is less true the younger the child and the higher the fever.

But fundamentally a child that has a fever and looks ok, probably is ok.

Learn to recognise a sick child as soon as you walk into the waiting room – even if they are not booked as your patient. A child who is pale and floppy and lying listlessly in their mother's arms is a worry. If they are too exhausted to cry, they are in serious trouble. And the reverse is also largely true.

A child that is active enough to get into trouble is probably not in trouble.

Whilst we rely on parents to give us an accurate description of how young Charlie's behaviour has changed in the past day or two, we need to also judge with our own eyes. If a child is running around the room pulling books off the shelf, sticking toys into the printer holes, and fingers into the power sockets, they are probably not seriously unwell.

On the other hand, as the resident in charge of paediatrics in a busy emergency department, my own guideline was "Any child who will let me do a lumbar puncture, needs a lumbar puncture." Whilst that isn't always the case, a child that unwell will probably need a prompt septic workup, preferably in hospital where results are quickly to hand.

For this reason, any time you invest in winning an infant or toddler's trust is valuable. No matter how busy we are, or how sick they look, you want to try and make the child trust you. And the best way to do that is to make them laugh. And often the best way to do that is to make the parent laugh first.

Whilst it's important to treat a child of any age as an autonomous individual, and centre them as the patient in the consultation, it's ok to start that process by focussing on the parent first, and gradually acclimatising Charlie to your presence, your voice and your behaviour.

For most infants and toddlers, I will often start by examining – very carefully and thoroughly – their mother's hands; palmar and dorsal; and test her pulse. If there is a cooperative older sibling, so much the better. Let's get them involved as well and normalise the physical exam. If Charlie brought a toy, examine his teddy-bear together with him. Let him wield the tongue depressor, and even a stethoscope. I often get three-year-olds to look in Mum's ears and maybe even get them to look in their own – put a speculum in their ear whilst they look through the otoscope in their hand! They never argue about the exam after that.

For slightly older children, if not too unwell, I have a different stratagem. I will often introduce myself with the child's name and demonstrate great confusion about who in the room is the child-patient, the parent, the doctor and whose name belongs to whom. This falls flat sometimes, but most three-year-olds find this hilarious and fall over themselves trying to explain "I'm the patient and my name is Charlie; that's the Daddy and his name is Sam and you're the doctor!", whilst I helplessly ask, "Then who is David?"

Fill your bucket with ways to examine children. If Charlie won't let you examine his abdomen, then ask him to examine himself whilst you put your hand on top to show him where to press and how deeply. Then ask to swap hands over with him pushing yours down. Learn some children's poetry by A.A. Milne and the latest songs by the Wiggles so you can recite them and sing them to and with your patients.

And always be alert for the child too unwell to protest.

CHAPTER 19

What Matters Most

Whether with money, time or both, patients aren't paying us just for the exalted honour of being in our esteemed company. Why do they do it? Primarily because they want an answer, a treatment, a cure.

The problem of course is that before you can fix a problem, you need to identify it and sometimes that takes time, and sometimes it's not possible at all. Our first job then (there seem to be a lot of things that are our first job) is to ensure the patient knows what is and isn't possible.

In most cases, patients are very happy with that. In my experience – perhaps because I am blessed with a reasonably health-literate population, perhaps because I have well-trained patients – most are happy to be part of a diagnostic and therapeutic process that takes time. Of course, some new patients do walk in with a 20-year unsolved pain or paraesthesia with the expectation that they will walk out with their symptoms cured. But the majority, whether new or established patients, come in wanting to see what you are going to do.

Sometimes the best management plan is to do nothing. Watchful waiting, seeing how a symptom or even disease evolves, allowing the natural history of a condition to declare itself, can be incredibly helpful. Indeed, it is one of the key features distinguishing hospital medicine from general practice. In hospital, the most expensive test you can order is "Nurse, keep this patient in bed. We'll come back tomorrow." That's a test that costs over $1000 a day!

But we use that test in general practice all the time. "Mr Brown – I don't think that spot is anything but let's watch it for four weeks and see what happens. If it's not gone by then, we will take it off." "Mrs Smith – here's an x-ray form. I think this is just a sprain, but if it's just as sore tomorrow, go over to radiology."

We use time for diagnosis, we use time for treatment, in a way that is impossible in hospitals.

Why do patients tolerate this? Because once they understand that you have their best interests at heart, they no longer demand instantaneous fixes. They are happy to pay for your expertise, even if that expertise says "I'm not quite sure."

How do they know that you have their best interests at heart? By the quality of your explanation of your thinking.

It is not essential to have the answer, but it is critical to have a plan.

A patient is relying on you to hold their hand and lead them on their health journey, whether for an acute problem or a chronic illness. You are not expected to know where every twist and turn on the road is – but you need to map out the general route and show them that you know the way.

We do this by giving patients an overview of what lies ahead, and then revising and filling that in as we go along. Patients – indeed people – are much more scared of the unknown than the known. Saying "Trust me" doesn't generate trust – it generates fear of what you aren't saying.

But saying "I'm not sure what the lump is. We're going to do an ultrasound. If it shows something, I know who to send you to. If the ultrasound shows nothing of concern, we will wait four weeks and if it still persists, we will use a two-week course of nolumpium. I don't want to prescribe that just yet, because of the possible side-effects", shows you are in perfect control of the situation, without having a clue what the lump is.

It's as important not to overshare information as it is to leave a patient hanging without an explanation. Rare is the patient who wants a full diagnostic algorithm regarding thyroid testing the day they come in with general fatigue. They just want to know you've thought of it. Most patients aren't interested in the layers of the abdomen that must be incised on the way to reaching the appendix.

It's also important to know what the patient already knows. As we discussed in Chapter 13, a patient who comes in with a lump is probably thinking about cancer, a patient who has a tremor is possibly worried about Parkinson's disease. If you don't mention these things, then from their perspective you haven't thought about them, and that means that your plan is inadequate.

Show the patient that you know the way and they will gladly follow your plan.

CHAPTER 20

The Robin Hood Clock

The number one complaint that patients make about GPs is that they were kept waiting too long. The number two complaint is that the GP didn't spend enough time with them!

Trying to create an appointment system that works is a fruitless task. Doctors aren't stupid – if there was a better method, we would have found it by now! The reason that doctors run late is that unlike lawyers, accountants and architects, most of our work is conducted in the appointment room, not in the back office. And we do our work back-to-back. But patients can come in with *anything!* It might be a repeat script; it might be an emotional breakdown. Unless the patient warns the booking staff of exactly what the problem is, and the system is flexible enough to move every other patient that day around, you will never have appointments of exactly the right length.

Even then, you don't know whether the patient booked in to discuss a spot has an obvious wart or a potential melanoma. It's not reasonable to expect patients to know that headache for three weeks takes much longer to assess than knee pain for three weeks.

What's been tried?

a) No appointments. This is how hospital outpatients and some general practice clinics used to run. No appointments, just show up on the designated day (hospitals) or the day you want to be seen (GPs) and be seen in turn – first come, first served. The afternoon session began at 2pm, so everyone would either arrive at 1pm hoping to be seen first, or they would arrive at the last permitted minute hoping that the crush before them had thinned. It resulted in crowded waiting rooms, grumpy patients, stressed receptionists and harassed doctors.

b) Appointment waves. Designating 1/3 of your patients to come at 2pm, another third at 3pm, and the final third at 4pm, was an effort to smooth out the flow. It still resulted in patients arriving early in the hope of reducing their waiting time by at least an hour, and generally got fuller toward the end of the session.

c) Fixed appointments with rigid times. This is the commonest way to see patients – 10 or 15 minute appointment slots. Patients book the time they want. The problem is that the patient before them might arrive late, have an obscure diagnosis, have multiple problems, burst into tears, or present without an appointment because chest pain doesn't respect scheduling.

d) Variable appointment lengths – where you educate patients to allow more time for a greater number or more complex problems or if they are chatty. Great in theory, but assumes patients have the literacy to know how long their appointments will take, and have the self-discipline to cut their own consult short if they are approaching their self-selected time limit. Good luck with that one!

e) Modified waves. In an effort to take the best of b and c, the modified wave system evolved. If you book patients at 9:00, 9:15 and 9:30, then should your first appointment run 5 minutes long and the second one 5 minutes short, you are back on track. But if the first one runs short and the second one overtime – you are five minutes late for every patient for the rest of the day.

Instead, if your book says 9:00, 9:10 and 9:30, then the second patient will typically wait just 5 minutes, or in the case the first patient runs over, the second will wait just 10 minutes. Your day will still be on track at 9:30. However if the first patient is the quick one and the second one takes longer – you've lost no time in your day.

The reality is that there isn't any perfect system because patients aren't pegs to be squeezed into appointment holes. So we need to find a way to

Steal time from the rich and give to the poor.

Some patients need and deserve more time. Some simple problems can be dealt with simply, without dragging out the consult to fill the time available. Our practice sums it up thus – we dedicate the time needed to the patient in front of us, whilst being aware of the patients sitting in the waiting room.

I am fully aware of the contradictions that I have now placed before you. Just as "He who hesitates is lost" and "Look before you leap" are both true, I hold that on the one hand we should wind up an appointment when it's appropriate to do so, even if there is theoretically time remaining, and yet in Chapter 8, I recommended that "at every consultation do one thing the patient didn't ask for".

You have to embrace the messiness of general practice.

CHAPTER 21

The Screams Of Silence

Given that patients are paying for the time they spend with us, there is an understandable tendency to want to prove to them that that time is being well spent. Taking a history, performing an exam are not just diagnostic, they are also performative. The patient can see that we are investing time in their welfare.

But sometimes the hardest and best work we do involves withdrawing into ourselves. It might be crafting a good referral letter. It might be reading a discharge summary or specialist letter and really thinking about the next steps. It might just be sitting and thinking deeply about what the patient has said.

But what is the patient doing whilst we are sitting and contemplating? What are they looking at and what are they thinking? (Actually, one of the best teaching techniques, now rarely used due to the stringencies of the Medical Records Act, is to videotape registrar consultations and play them back during a tutorial. Watching the doctor-patient interaction is invaluable. Watching what a patient does whilst the GP is out of the room or is staring at the computer screen is priceless!)

One way to deal with an awkward silence is to mutter. When writing a letter, you can check key points whilst typing. If you are reading a letter or summary or complex radiology report, it's quite effective to just mutter out the key words, to give the patient a sense of what you are reading which you will later synthesise.

We will meet Dr Les Segal in Chapter 25. One of his rules is to review the patient's file including past history, family history, recent presentations, results and specialist/hospital letters before you call the patient into the room. He is right! This minimises silence, maximises effectiveness and shows your mastery of the patient to the patient. It may be reasonable to review points of a patient's history or ask if anything has changed, but the patient wants to feel that they are important enough to you that you particularly remember them as an individual.

Re-reading the notes before you start will not just remind you of your thought process and where you are up to in the diagnostic or management arc, but also allows you to refresh yourself on your human touchpoints. If you jot down a social history note about the patient's upcoming grandchild, or their daughter's graduation, you have a beautiful entry point to the consultation that patients will value as personal. If you stumble across that note whilst browsing in front of the patient it comes across as formulaic.

But strictly Medicare doesn't cover time spent without the patient in front of you, and you can spend an awful lot of your day in unpaid reading whilst patients get frustrated by being kept waiting in another room. Muttering therefore fills the painful silence that develops while the patient is watching you review consultations, investigations and correspondence.

On the other hand, sometimes the best way to get a patient to speak is to say nothing. If you reach an awkward pause in a consult, rather than ask another question, it may be effective to sit still and say nothing. Nature abhors a vacuum, and most people abhor silence, particularly if it is not with a close friend. If you don't speak – chances are, they will. And often how they lead off tells you a lot more than a hundred questions you might ask which can lead in irrelevant directions.

But if you fill that silence with muttering trite words then you kill the silence that builds rapport and generates trust.

Sometimes for good and sometimes for bad – muttering kills silence.

Perhaps one exception to this is when you are deeply thinking about what your next steps are – formulating your differential list, considering which tests and in which order, or the pros and cons of various medications. It's helpful to cultivate a "thinking face", that lets the patient know that you aren't just daydreaming about that night's dinner recipe.

And of course a simple option is to let the patient know – "I'm just going to go quiet for a minute while I think."

Words matter. Muttering matters. Silence matters. Knowing which to use when matters.

CHAPTER 22

Welcome back!

In your hospital years, you almost certainly did a rotation in the Emergency Department. Recall that if a patient attended ED and came back a day or so later, someone looked down their nose at you and implied that somehow you failed.

But in general practice, when a patient comes back – we like that! We call it continuity of care, and that's a win!

Why? What is it about general practice that makes seeing a patient more than once not just acceptable, but desirable?

Why do we review a patient?

There needs to be more than one answer to this, because there is more than one type of review. And the reason for that is that is there are fundamentally three reasons patients present.

First – an episode of acute care. This is the ED model. A patient has a symptom or a sign and wants to know why and wants to see it gone. It might be a runny nose, a changing mole, a dull ache in the knee, a crushing pain in the chest, a month of sadness.

All chronic illnesses start with an initial and therefore acute presentation, but clearly not all first presentations go on to be chronic illnesses.

Acute medicine isn't limited to a single visit or a single symptom. The whole point of taking a history and doing an examination is to gather the strands of hidden data. If a patient knew that night sweats, loss of weight, change in bowel habit and a constant rib pain are all related – they would present all those symptoms to you in a single package during their initial narrative of why they have come in today.

It's the symptoms they didn't realise are significant, or didn't think you wanted to hear about that you need to elicit. And of course, examination often finds things patients weren't aware of – deep tenderness, a mass, lung crackles, fundal changes, pan-systolic murmurs.

If you have no answer, you have a journey to travel and that includes investigations, possibly specialist referral but above all review. You are seeing if the symptoms or signs are evolving. You are seeing how the patient's response to the symptoms and signs is evolving.

We review a patient to reassure them – either that there is nothing significantly wrong, so there is nothing to worry about, or there may be something wrong but they are safe in our hands, and so there is nothing to worry about.

We also review the patient to reassure ourselves – either that there is nothing of deep concern, even though we don't know what is going on, or that there is something serious, but that we are in control and have done all that is necessary or reasonable or possible.

The second reason patients present is for ongoing management of chronic illness. This might be a three-monthly diabetes review or a BP check. It might be a regular script renewal for a patient with stable asthma. It might be a six-monthly review of depression.

The easy thing to do in a chronic illness review is to review the disease. Lungs sound OK? Here's your puffer. Weight is a touch up, HbA1c is a touch down? Here's your script and a blood test form for three months' time.

The more worthwhile approach to chronic illness is to review the patient. What complications have arisen? What might evolve before the next visit? What's the big picture – is the weight creeping up, up, up over a three-year period – and now it's 8 kg more than when we started? What are the health benefits of losing 5kg, and what obstacles prevent that happening?

The difficulty with managing chronic illness is that in the absence of definitive cure there is no obvious end-goal. With an acute illness we strive primarily, or at least initially, for a diagnosis, a label. Once we have that we work towards a cure.

But with chronic illness we know that it's there forever and what we strive for is control, perhaps remission, deferral of complications. So it's easy to take the easy route and only do the needful, rather than actively thinking where we can add value to a patient's life and health at every interaction.

In that sense, chronic disease is more similar to preventative health than to acute medicine. A mole check, a pap smear, a home medication review are rarely going to find something unexpected. But they are part of a process of establishing an ongoing relationship with patients that makes them comfortable and confident to come to us with anything.

The third reason patients see us is for preventative healthcare, whether initiated by them or by us. This is the epitome of review for review's sake. An annual checkup is almost limitless in scope – weight, girth, blood pressure, blood tests, pap smear, immunisations, bowel check, skin check, mental health, diet, exercise, sleep, relationships, stressors, life goals, family and social history ...

Such reviews reassure the patient and reassure us. We can't travel a journey with patients unless we spend time with them. Preventative health is not a march to a destination – it's a meandering stroll that hopefully gets you nowhere!

You don't need to be a GP to check a blood pressure. A nurse or physician's assistant can do that just as well as we can. But it is the regular check-ups and check-ins that we do that means when we say "It's time to start medication" the patient will believe, accept and act.

Reviewing patients is the essence of the journey we travel with them as their GPs.

CHAPTER 23

Known Unknowns

An expert knows more and more about less and less, till they know virtually everything about almost nothing.

Being a generalist involves knowing a lot about some things, a fair bit about most things, and at least something about everything. That little might just be knowing that you know nothing about it other than it exists.

You will often get stuck when a patient presents with an odd rash, bizarre symptoms, unusual presentations. As you develop experience, (and more importantly, confidence in your experience), you'll be able to say one of two things to such a patient:

"I don't know what it is – but I'm comfortable that it isn't something serious." (As we discussed in Chapter 12 - Tell the patient what it's not). "Something this bizarre just doesn't fit with anything. I think we can wait and see if it goes away by itself or worsens and declares itself in some other way"; or

"I don't know what it is – but it certainly seems like it's something. What I do know is who the right person is to tell us. I'd like you to see Professor Supersmarts. Here's what I'd like you to do before you go, so that she has the maximum information when you first see her."

Rare diseases in general practice are surprisingly common. If your practice has 5000 patients, you will probably have in that cohort people with Marfan's syndrome, Ehlers-Danlos disease and Huntington's disease. Somebody had to diagnose them initially – and that can be you when the next one presents.

We come out of university and hospital years with a head stuffed full of knowledge that gradually dissipates because our rare diseases muscle is so rarely exercised. Gradually our alertness to the obscuroma fades. Our task is to keep refreshing the brain database with those rarities, through case discussion with colleagues, journals and online quizzes, education days and specialist lectures.

Some years ago, I was consulted by a patient late on a Saturday afternoon. She had been my patient a decade or more earlier but had moved on to another practice. But she wanted me – that weekend – to find the cause of the tiredness that she had suffered for several years but was progressively worsening, and that no other doctor had been able to diagnose or treat. Of note, she had diabetes under the care of an endocrinologist.

Doing the right thing I took a solid history and teased out there was some weight loss! Among the many negative answers, when I asked about diet, she agreed that she might have a bit of salt craving!! With a bit of nudging, her husband agreed her colour may be a little more tanned than normal!!!

"Oh wow!", I thought, "Not only have I found an elusive case of Addison's disease – I have found it in a patient who sees an endocrinologist and he's missed it! Which of course makes perfect sense. In this case, he is the "GP" seeing the patient three monthly for diabetes review and not alert to thinking about the insidious onset of other conditions. I am the "specialist" seeing her with fresh eyes for a second opinion, and therefore more tuned in to thinking about the unusual."

Indeed, I am alert to the possibility of Addison's disease, having missed diagnosing a case in my early general practice days, though I did at least recognise her as significantly unwell and sent her to a general physician. He deservedly got the credit for the diagnosis before referring her on to an endocrinologist. And I swore that I would never miss another case of Addison's, and that I wouldn't retire until I found one to make up for the one I missed.

So with a bit of excitement I tracked down my patient's diabetes specialist then and there and relayed my findings, and asked if he wanted to admit her immediately for testing. It was clear from the boredom in his voice that he thought I was an overreacting idiot wasting his time on a Saturday afternoon. Or was I perhaps detecting a bit of defensiveness that a GP had outdiagnosed him? In any event he agreed to arrange an ACTH stimulation test.

I cannot begin to express how angry I was when the test came back normal!

So here is a case where there was no rare diagnosis, and I wasn't the hero I could have been, nor did I get a story to tell at medical dinners for decades to come. (Though I do tell the story about how I don't have the story!).

Nonetheless, when I reflect on that weekend, I remain proud that I practiced solid medicine – remaining alert to the possibility of the rarity.

And it emphasised that

You don't need to know every diagnosis. But you need to know that there are ones you don't know.

I will spare you the horror of my porphyria story.

CHAPTER 24

Doctor Knows Best

There are certain mantras that become so ingrained in our student years and early careers that they become articles of truth regardless of how true they actually are. So forgive me if I try to shake up one of the key things you have no doubt had impressed upon you.

There is no evidence for Evidence-Based Medicine.

Of course medicine is based on science. I do not for one moment minimise the importance of the basic and applied clinical sciences to good medicine. Nor do I disparage in any way the centrality of keeping up with the literature of advances in healthcare. Indeed, at my graduation, the speaker pointed out that after six years of university, our heads were stuffed full of the latest medical knowledge ... but that within five years, half of what we were taught would be wrong. And there was no way of knowing which half.

Thus, over the years, many clearcut, well established medical facts are no more. Smoking doesn't relax you. Using long-acting beta-agonists for baseline asthma treatment and inhaled corticosteroids for flareups isn't the way to go.

Digitalis has been used for heart failure, for atrial fibrillation, for AF rate control but not rhythm control, rhythm control but not rate control, failure in AF but not in other conditions and so on. Ipratropium was first line for asthma, second line for asthma, first line in kids but not adults, first line for adults but not kids, first line for COPD but not asthma and not useful at all.

I don't mock these changes – the most important aspect of scientific method is to be open to new information. But the corollary of that is not to be wedded to old information as absolutely and invariably true.

The problem with Evidence-Based Medicine is that the evidence it is based upon is usually inapplicable. As GPs we are all busy, and over time we read less and less basic research material. But if you do pick up a paper to read the details of a study, before deciding how much your practice will change as a result, turn to the most important part of any clinical trial – the exclusion criteria.

The issue is that many, if not most trials, exclude the complicated, multimorbid patients that make up the bulk of our day. They need to – such patients represent a multitude of variables that can't be corrected for making study interpretation difficult, and they represent a major risk of side-effects, interactions or complications that drug companies and researchers would desperately like to avoid. But those are the very patients for whom we are most seeking answers!

There has never been a true trial of EBM. If there were, it would compare the outcomes generated by a medical student with a stack of guidelines against the outcomes of a GP with 20 years' experience.

In fact, for the sake of your own career, you had better hope that EBM isn't valid. Because if it is, a nurse or medical student armed with ChatGPT or the latest AI, is going to be much better at patient outcomes than you are. I hold little fear of this. AI is good at searching and synthesising the facts of EBM, but at this stage at least is poor at perspective and context – not what is going on, but what is going on with **this** patient at **this** time.

I may well be wrong, but I think knowledge with compassion (see Chapter 61) is something AI will never be able to achieve. As GPs, we must begin with deep knowledge, but we must end with deep empathy and communication.

What EBM does provide is a basis for your consideration. What EBM doesn't do – and what a skilled GP like you has been trained to do – is actually think!

CHAPTER 25

Step right up!

Our clinic is now in its third location, having started in a house, moved to a shopping centre and is now in a purpose-built facility. The second site, in a shopping centre, consisted of two shops one behind the other, so it was basically a waiting room at the front, a long central corridor and doors off either side.

The shop fitter used one type of vinyl for the waiting area, and another pattern of vinyl along the corridor.

A couple of years after we opened the clinic we were joined by my teacher, friend and mentor Dr Les Segal, who came to us after 30 years of solo general practice. Les is a deeply knowledgeable and caring doctor, an exceptional teacher but above all a wonderful, warm human being.

Apart from the large cohort of patients who were willing to travel 40 minutes each way to continue seeing him, he rapidly developed a following of patients with complex medical conditions. He was particularly liked by elderly patients for whom he has near-infinite patience and interest.

It took some time before I noticed that Les was doing something very odd. The rest of us would walk down the corridor to call in our next patient. We'd get to the end of the corridor, stand next to the reception desk at the edge of the waiting room and call our next patient. We would politely wait until someone stood up and approached us. We would acknowledge them, turn and lead them down the corridor to our room. Very nice.

But Les wouldn't call a patient's name. He would scan the waiting room till he saw his patient and then walk up to them with hand extended. If they were frail, he would help them to their feet, or at least greet them and stand patiently next to them whilst they stood up and grabbed their walker. If warranted, he would gently guide them toward his room. If not, he would merely exchange pleasantries whilst walking alongside them down the corridor.

If he didn't recognise the patient by name or it was a new patient, he would, as we all did, call out the patient's name but at the first sign of someone stirring out of their chair, walk up to them and repeat the warm welcome above.

It seemed very, very odd and it took me a little while to realise what was going on. The rest of us would come to a hard stop on the line where the vinyl changed colour. Like germs that are unable to jump over the red line at the entrance to the sterile area of theatre, it seemed we were afraid of being sullied if we set foot in the waiting room. Once I realised that this is what we were doing it was amusing to see how millimetre perfectly doctors would instinctively place their feet just before but never over the razor thin join between two coloured pieces of plastic flooring.

Segal's manoeuvre as I call it (but can only type with the grace of spell check and auto correct), taught me that the consultation begins not with the opening question, but with the first glance between patient and doctor. First impressions matter not just on first meeting but at every encounter. If we greet our patient with a scowl or sense of hurry, then we are saying that we don't care or don't have time for them today, even if we've seen them satisfactorily for years previously.

In contrast, going up to a patient with a smile, a sense of recognition, a hand extended to shake says much louder than words "I am so pleased to see you again. I can't wait to continue our journey together."

If you are in a busy practice, I urge you to spend 10 minutes either at the reception desk or even better sitting in the waiting room. Watch patients as they arrive, sit, wait and wonder when will they be called. Watch the doctors as they approach from the consulting wing. Do they call from the doorway? Do they enter the waiting room? Or do they execute a perfect Segal's manoeuvre and

Go up to the patient in the waiting room.

Then see if you can detect a difference in the way each consultation begins.

Perhaps this habit of calling people from a distance is a protective mechanism we develop from hospital outpatient clinics, where we usually do not know the patient, and so calling out their name like a railway station announcer is necessary. Entering a hospital outpatient waiting room can feel like walking into a dark laneway outside a sticky-floor pub in a seedy area of an unfamiliar town – lots of strangers giving you shifty looks as to who you are and what you are doing there.

And truthfully, the larger a practice is, the harder it is to know who everyone in the waiting room is and see them as good acquaintances. Particularly of course as a registrar just getting to know the patient base.

But I strongly encourage you to spend a couple of days deliberately alternating between doing and not doing Segal's manoeuvre and seeing what a difference it makes to the start of your consultations.

CHAPTER 26

Root Cause Analysis

One of the great learning experiences of my medical student days were the lectures by the late Dr John Colvin, ophthalmologist, at the Royal Victorian Eye and Ear Hospital. As reluctant as we were to be in the city at 8am on a Saturday morning, ophthalmology was appallingly taught at university and general hospitals, but brilliantly taught by this pedagogic genius.

This was the only opportunity throughout our training when students from University of Melbourne and Monash University came together, and Dr Colvin played up the rivalry to no end. This alone kept us engaged for no one wished to let down their side by answering a lobbed question incorrectly. To top it off, he engaged a musician to stand at the back of the hall, and whenever he was about to make a salient point, would signal for a trumpet blast to shake us back to alertness so that we wouldn't miss the pearl he was about to impart.

Or rather than pearl – gold. Because, long before there was an Idiot's Guide to Everything, he managed to condense all of what was necessary and practical in ophthalmology for non-ophthalmologists into the iconic "35 Golden Eye Rules". If you are not familiar with these, please search for them, print them and memorise them.

The second of these rules is a quote by Dr Thomas McCrae "More mistakes in medicine are made by not looking than not knowing." Whilst Dr Colvin was referring to illumination, dilation of the pupil and practice in fundoscopy, it applies to all aspects of clinical medicine. "If you don't put your finger in it – you put your foot in it" and "There are only two reasons not to do a PR exam – the patient has no anus or the doctor has no finger" are two further aphorisms about the importance of actually actively looking for pathology.

Leaving an obvious foreign body to be found so that candidates miss the second one is a classic trick case in the Fellowship clinical exam! I recall hearing of a woman with uterine didelphys and a baby in each. Did nobody notice two cervices when doing her Pap smears? As Sherlock Holmes said "You see, but you do not observe." We notice what we expect and do not see all that there is.

However there is a greater reason for missing clues in history, signs on exam and solutions to problems. Dr Clare Turner added a significant advance to the already profound thought above and wrote:

More mistakes in medicine are made by not looking than not knowing, but most mistakes are made by not caring.

So true. Because, whilst on the one hand, Turner's law takes in all of Drs McCrae and Colvin's idea – someone who doesn't care enough to even look is certainly going to miss things, Dr Turner goes a step further and points out that the whole underpinning of good general practice is that we care enough about our patients to always – always – do more than the minimum. We ask another question, we examine a little more slowly and carefully, we take a little more time in explaining, we think a little deeper, we ask colleagues a little more often.

We need to care for two reasons. First, it protects us from making simple, preventable, obvious mistakes. Not caring implies being careless!

Second, our patients don't want skilled robots. They want a doctor for whom they matter. As (possibly) President Theodore Roosevelt famously said "Nobody cares how much you know until they know how much you care."

Turner's law encapsulates all these ideas. It's the perfect bridge from being a decent human to being a great doctor.

CHAPTER 27

Shadow Jumping

Clothes maketh the man. Never judge a book by its cover. You're never too old to learn. You can't teach an old dog new tricks. Absence makes the heart grow fonder. Out of sight, out of mind.

There is no end to proverbs, aphorisms and sayings that contradict each other. I've done it already (eg Chapters 16 and 17, Chapters 8 and 20) and am about to do it again.

As a GP it's hard to find pathology because we are often lulled into a false sense of security. In ED, most patients are unwell. In specialist practice, most patients have been triaged by their GP, so that only the sicker ones are seen. But in general practice we see the sick, the well, the worried, the wondering. We treat patients, not diseases, so often there is no pathology other than a patient's concern.

The corollary is that we need to work harder than specialists to find pathology. When you know there is a high chance there is something wrong, you are on the alert for subtle changes. If most of the time that's a waste of time because the patient is perfectly well, it's easy to fall into the habit of rushed history, perfunctory exam and minimal thought.

The reverse is to always live in fear of what you are missing. It's easy to prove the presence of disease. It's much harder to convincingly demonstrate there is nothing there. Proof of absence is notoriously difficult – ask any atheist!

So the difficulty for GPs is working out when to go hunting for a disease that is unlikely to be there, and how far to go down the path of investigation looking for increasingly obscure diagnoses even when nothing is driving this other than a vague sense of unease.

Pay great heed to that feeling. Your instinct is honed by experience, even if you don't remember it. And Connoley's Law (Chapter 29) teaches us how important it is not to stress but to act.

Nonetheless, at some point you have to stop. No matter how hard you hunt for snarks, you aren't going to find one. At some point you will frustrate the patient and exhaust yourself, or perhaps exhaust the patient and frustrate yourself.

At that point stop and remember –

There are rarely sharks in swimming pools.

Awareness that the uncommon exists is critical to safe general practice. Fear of the unlikely is anathema to good general practice.

Every GP has to find their own comfort zone between doing too little and doing too much. But if you are presenting a case to your supervisor, your colleague or yourself and find yourself saying "I know this is ridiculously unlikely but ...", then you are probably right.

CHAPTER 28

A Pointed Question

We spend a lot of time talking about opening a consultation. Many pages (and Chapter 5 of this book) have been written about what exactly our opening words should be.

We speak much less often about how to close a consultation. What is the best way to end a visit?

The biggest trap, that I fall into far more often than I should given my experience, is to conclude a consultation by asking "Is there anything else?" That is a recipe for starting a whole new consultation when I'm already running overtime on this one, and unacceptably late for my next one!

There are a number of other closing methods that are sometimes recommended. One is to always book the next appointment. I remember once talking to the founder of a highly entrepreneurial physiotherapy chain who said "We never discharge a patient. We always book them for the next visit."

Perhaps because it's not my world I think that's overservicing by physios. But in the dental world it is considered quite normal to book the next treatment appointment – or series of appointments – when their need is recognised, and to book a preventative dental health check up in six or twelve months if no active treatment is needed.

Since, as GPs, we do a mix of acute, chronic and preventative care, there is no reason not to, and plenty of reasons why we should, adopt the same model. There's never enough time for proper preventative health – it's mostly just a little add on we throw in when we are running on time. I don't want to presume your abilities, but checking on diet, exercise, sleep, rest, smoking, caffeine, alcohol, drugs, recreation, screening based on family, social and personal risk factors, reviewing mental health, family dynamics, sense of purpose and lifeplan for the next ten years is something I struggle to fit-in in the final three minutes of a consultation.

My typical closing line – which I hate myself for every time I say it – is "I'll see you when you need me." But the truth is we can provide so much more care for patients if we proactively see them rather than just reactively!

The main downside of this strategy is the loss of appointment availability for more acute needs. I have no great solution to that other than managing your appointment book with a series of on the day, on the week, doctor only to book and anyone can prebook appointments.

Another closing consultation error is to follow the classic advice of having the patient explain back to you the whole history, diagnosis, prognosis and management plan. Whilst this is ideal if there is unlimited time, it can come close to doubling the length of the consultation, comes across as condescending a lot of the time, and embarrasses patients who aren't terribly health literate.

More appropriately I think, is to ask a patient if they are clear on the plan, and if they are happy (or at least comfortable) with the plan. We need to be careful that this question is asked genuinely, for it is much easier for a patient to nod yes, than to say "Actually – no!" If there is any sense that you won't be happy with the negative answer, you won't get it – in which case there was no point in asking the question.

This brings me to my final point and to universalise that. If (as embarrassingly I have done) you ask a question to which you already know the answer ("Oh ... your wife died yesterday – how are you?") – why are you asking that question? If you ask a question but are cornering the patient into giving you a specific answer ("I've explained this to you twice ... do you need me to go over it again?") – why are you asking that question? And if you are asking a question, but you don't really want to hear the answer ("Now that we've dealt with your six main problems, is there anything else I can do for you today?") – then why are you asking that question?

Lawyers are taught never to ask a witness in court a question if they don't already know the answer. We of course need to do that to take a history. But

Every question must have a purpose.

Every question should be asked with a genuine point and the answer genuinely heard.

There is a well-known mantra that before you order a test – ask yourself, what will you do if the test is positive? What will you do if the test is negative? If the answer is the same – why are you doing the test?

The same applies to the questions you ask!

CHAPTER 29

Sweet Dreams

As a registrar, I was assessed every six weeks with formal feedback forms on history taking, examination technique, clinical reasoning and understanding of the context of general practice. I did ok, never brilliantly, on all of those.

But where I scored really badly was on "tolerance of uncertainty". I'm about as Type A as you can get. I love maths. Ticking a correct answer is my dopamine hit, equivalent to hitting a mini-jackpot on a poker-machine. Getting an answer wrong is disappointing ... but not knowing the answer is frustrating beyond belief.

Over the years I've gotten better at dealing with the not knowing. Much of the time, it doesn't matter if we have an exact answer, as long as we are travelling in the right direction.

Every doctor will have their own limits of ease or discomfort. Whilst it's important to develop an acceptance that not everything can, or even needs to be known, you also need to respect your own level of anxiety and concern.

GP medical educators hammer home to registrars the importance of dealing with uncertainty. But we only see you in the clinic. We aren't listening to your internal dialogue when you have finished your day, yet take the patient home with you inside your head.

And so I recommend you live by Connoley's Law –

If you are going to lose sleep over it, do something about it.

Taught to me by Dr Grant Connoley, an experienced GP, excellent teacher and a master of letting go, it summarises that you need to finish your day with a clear head and a cleared agenda, and not spend the next 12 hours unproductively second guessing yourself.

You can't send every vague abdominal pain for immediate ultrasound. You can't send every sprained ankle for an x-ray - "just in case". If you send every headache to ED with a letter asking for an MRI, you might even find yourself somehow blacklisted.

But neither can you spend every night in tears or poring over textbooks looking for all the things you coulda, shoulda, woulda done if only ...

As we have discussed in Chapter 22, there are many reasons to review a patient. Your own serenity is one of them. If it will give you eight hours undisturbed rest, invest 5 minutes at the end of your day calling that patient you saw in the morning with asthma, just to be sure that they haven't deteriorated as the sun started to set. If need be, stay back 30 minutes and see them once more, or arrange some prednisolone, or send them to ED.

General practice is all about balancing competing needs. In Chapter 41 we will discuss the tension between being perfect and being good enough. Here we deal with the inherent issue of staying sane in general practice by not obsessing, and at the same time accepting that some things can't be accepted.

You will need to find your own middle ground and path. It will get easier with time and experience. Above all it will get easier with reflection. Think about whether you are investigating or treating the patient, their family ... or yourself. There's nothing wrong with that, as long as you are honest with yourself (and the patient) that that is what you are doing.

It's possible that some patients will think you are over-investigating or over-reviewing to squeeze out another consult and a few more dollars. That's ok – they will find a doctor who is more chill. Others will be grateful that you are looking a little deeper, or "better safe than sorry". Eventually you will fill your day with patients who appreciate that your worry levels are not too hot, not too cold, but just right for them.

CHAPTER 30

Heart And Head

There is an old joke that asks what is the difference between involvement and commitment? Well – when you eat bacon and eggs, the chicken is involved, but the pig is committed.

The common thread through several recent chapters is to understand the equal but differing roles of the patient and the doctor in the consultation. We walk into the room with different knowledge, experience, values, expectations. But mostly the difference is in the degree of involvement and commitment.

For a patient, every consultation is a cry for help – sometimes louder or softer, sometimes more or less desperate, sometimes more or less clearly defined. But a patient doesn't spend the time or money to see a doctor if they don't feel there is something wrong.

The doctor on the other hand must first and foremost work out whether there is something wrong. If there is – what is it, how will we find it and how do we treat it? And if there is nothing wrong, then there most certainly is something wrong – else why does the patient feel as they do?

In other words, the patient walks in with a feeling about their illness. The role of the doctor is to think about the problem, but also to think about the patient's feelings. How you handle the consultation, how much the patient perceives you have involved yourself in their unique symptoms, case, problem, life, will determine how they feel when they walk out. If they don't feel you have given them adequate time and consideration – if they don't feel you have truly thought about them, then they will leave disappointed, and almost certainly no better.

In brief –

The doctor does the thinking; the patient does the feeling.

Our thinking must be about both the illness – clinically – and about the patient – empathically. Neither alone is enough.

Knowledge without empathy is heartless; empathy (by a doctor) without knowledge is vacuous.

And so in a tangle of spirals and circles, they have to let us know why they feel uneasy and we have to think about the cause. We have to think about the patient's feelings, and patients have to let us know how they feel about our thinking. We need to care about the patient's dis-ease, and they need to think that we know what we are doing.

Remember our role is to lead and guide. If you find yourself so immersed in the patient's feelings that you are losing sight of the destination to which the patient should be heading, then you are being compassionate and a wonderful friend, but you may not be fulfilling your role as the health professional in the room.

But when you give a patient confidence in your knowledge and your care, they walk out of the room a little brighter, a little straighter, a little less burdened. A patient should always feel better when they leave a consultation than when they walked in.

CHAPTER 31

Past, Present And Future

The great contract-bridge player Benito Garozzo had a saying that in every deal a player should ask him or herself "What is the point of the hand?" In other words – rather than just make an automatic, standard bid or play of the cards, a player must identify what is the fundamental issue at hand.

The same applies to consultations. When a patient walks in, it is standard and relatively easy to take a history, conduct an exam, develop a list of differential diagnoses, order some tests, establish a management plan and farewell the patient.

What is much harder is to ask deeper questions, though that is what distinguishes a satisfactory consultation from a great one. Sometimes this is called "peeling the onion" – removing the layers of the presentation to get to the real heart of the consultation.

In some cases the patient knows what lies at the heart of the matter. They present their "ticket of entry" – starting with one problem when really they want to discuss another.

Some examples. A young man presents asking about a mole that is obviously benign, even to the lay person. Dig a little deeper and you may find concerns about a penile rash or a first episode of erectile dysfunction that was too embarrassing for him to bring up.

Or an elderly woman asking for a general checkup when she really wants to know whether she has dementia because this week she blanked out on the name of one of her grandchildren.

A more subtle form of peeling the onion is when the patient themselves is not aware of the deeper issues – but based on our experience we are. We think about both the triggers for a consultation and about the consequences.

A patient being bullied at work wants to make a Workcover claim. Fair enough – they are entitled to do so and may well even receive compensation. But in the majority of these consultations, I will preface the management by asking what the end game is. Because usually what the patient really wants is admission by the employer that they have been mistreated, and some form of sincere apology. Instead, if they enter into a litigious process, everyone's positions will become entrenched, each party's lawyers will warn against making any concessions, the case will proceed through several rounds of litigation and, in most cases, settle on the steps of court just before the trial proper begins. The victim will indeed receive a settlement. But after 2 or 3 years of legal manoeuvring they will not get the thing that they actually most want - acknowledgment of their feelings. And even if they obtain a court judgement and financial compensation, it is usually a hollow-feeling victory.

We don't have to talk them out of taking on the legalistic path. But a big part of our job is letting patients know what are the likely destinations of the train they are choosing to get on. They should be well informed before they buy that ticket.

Peeling back the layers of a consultation takes time, practice and the willingness of the patient to explore. Seeing into the future takes professional and life experience.

Some consultations don't need this. But almost always you will be serving the patient well if you ask yourself these two questions.

What came before? What comes after?

What came before? Because patients present to you for a reason. And they also don't present - for a reason. So always ask yourself - and frequently ask the patient - Why are they here ***today***? Why are they ***here*** today?

Why didn't they come yesterday or wait until tomorrow? ("You've had this pain for 3 months - why didn't you come a month ago? Why can't you put up with it for another month?")

Why are they seeing you and not their usual GP? Why are they seeing a doctor and not a dentist, physiotherapist, naturopath or lawyer? Why are they asking you and not their parent, child, friend or colleague?

Naturally, these should never be accusatory or smarmy questions. They are there to explore what lies underneath the symptoms.

A frequent example is the younger middle-aged man who comes in asking for "just a checkup". It's perhaps presumptuous to begin the consultation by asking "Why did your wife send you in today?" but it's accurate often enough to make you seem like a mind-reader! In my experience, when a 45 year old man presents for the first time for "just a checkup", it's been triggered either by something on the news (e.g. when Shane Warne died at the age of 52, we were flooded with middle aged men wanting heart checks) or by the heart attack of a close friend. And often it is the wife who insists upon (and books) the appointment.

Indeed, if a wife attends an appointment with her husband, you can be fairly certain that she is the patient – he is merely the presenting appendage.

What comes after? Because the consultation is a beginning, not an end.

Where will the unwell patient go? To the emergency department? Then will you write a letter or make a phone call? Are they going home? Then what if things deteriorate? When should they call you? (Are you available overnight – will you give your phone number to the patient?) If you want them to go to ED if things worsen, are you providing a letter to that effect for them to take with them overnight?

Does your patient have the language skills, confidence and wherewithal – given that they are acutely unwell – to make a timely appointment with the specialist – or do they need you to advocate for them to get an urgent appointment. Will they be fobbed off by the specialist's secretary?

Here's another example. A single mother brings one of her 3-year-old twins to see you with a straightforward history of croup, which began the night before. You can give the mum a script for prednisolone and congratulate yourself on your accurate diagnosis and management.

But think a bit deeper. Croup typically gets worse on nights two and three. What will mum do if the child gets worse? Can she call you? Would you go and assess the child at 3 am? If not – where should that mother and child go? And if you are really on your game, you will tell her now – at 4pm – to make arrangements for the other twin to either sleep out that night, or have someone on standby, so that if she and the patient do need to go to hospital in the middle of the night, she doesn't have to worry about the sibling's care.

A final example – your longstanding 25-year-old patient comes in for her contraceptive pill script before embarking that weekend on her 12-month volunteer role in a remote part of Africa. You've previously arranged all her vaccines, discussed water hygiene and bite prophylaxis, told her to travel with Australian made condoms and remembered today to do her first cervical screening test. But have you clarified how you will communicate the results to her if there is an abnormality? Did she leave an international number? Is it OK to email confidential results? Can you speak to her mother?

It's exhausting to always think about what came before and what comes after, what are the causes and what are the consequences. If you don't think about these things, you may still feel you are doing a good job. If you do think about them, you will realise just how hard it is to do a great job, and how satisfying it is when you do.

CHAPTER 32

On Silent Dogs

In Chapter 14 we discussed that abnormal results can often be found in healthy people. Not every pathology test that lies outside the reference range needs following up or even commenting on to your patient.

Is the reverse true? Are there completely normal results that should worry you? The answer – fairly obviously from the fact that I asked the question! – is of course. Sometimes, because when everything is normal you still don't know what's going on. And sometimes, because context is everything.

I tend, mostly, to be a "she'll be right, let's just wait and see" kind of doctor. Which is why I love spending time with doctors I respect who are more focussed on following up relatively minor abnormalities. I try to understand their thought process – why are they worried when I wouldn't be; and what will it take for them to accept that no further action is needed.

We should always consider the worst-case scenario – what could be going on here that is really bad. But having thought about it doesn't mean we need to obsessively hunt for it. We can, after all, sometimes let sleeping dogs lie.

Which is why I learned a valuable lesson from Dr Les Segal (Chapter 25) who presented a case at our clinical meeting. A middle-aged woman presented with tiredness of no obvious cause. History was unrevealing, examination was normal and all her blood tests were completely within normal limits.

I suspect I might have left further investigations there. There are lots of reasons for tiredness that aren't physical.

But Les was far from satisfied. He didn't just look at her results – he compared them to all her previous tests. And lo and behold – her ferritin, completely normal at 35, had been 200 less than a year earlier. Checking her haemoglobin showed that it too had gone from 150 g/l to 120 g/l. In other words – both tests had fallen from normal to normal, but in the context of the previous results these unremarkable numbers were highly significant.

Les sent the patient for a colonoscopy, which found an early colonic adenocarcinoma. The patient had a great outcome, Les had a great teaching story and I learned the importance of Segal's Law:

No ferritin or FBE is complete without looking at previous results.

Our previous chapter was about considering the context of the patient's life – What came before? Here we extend that to the realm of pathology – What results came before? Whilst haemoglobin and ferritin are the common examples of change that matters, I've learned to apply Segal's law in multiple other contexts.

Consider a steadily falling MCV as often the earliest sign of impending anaemia. An HbA1c that is creeping upwards over 12 months is screaming at you "Do something – more diet, more exercise or more medication, but don't pretend I will get better by myself." A falling eGFR might be benignly age related, or might be the sign that borderline hypertension needs much more than just annual checking.

When we weigh a patient, we don't just record it in that day's progress notes. We put it in the "height and weight module" of our software so that we can instantly compare today to yesterday, last month and last year.

A famous Sherlock Holmes mystery is solved because the dog didn't bark in the nighttime. Sometimes we let sleeping dogs lie – but sometimes we need to find out why they are softly snarling.

CHAPTER 33

The One With The Gold Makes The Rules

A long overdue movement in medicine is the notion of involving patients in all aspects of their own care. A common term for this is Shared Decision Making (SDM) – the notion that the doctor's role is to provide information to and collaborate with the patient but not to decide for them.

Indeed, this fits neatly with the primary meaning of the word "doctor" which comes from the Latin word meaning teacher. Thus a doctor of philosophy is someone with enough knowledge of a subject to teach the topic not just from a practical day-to-day perspective, but with enough wisdom to provide insight into the philosophical basis of the field, be it chemistry, anthropology or economics.

Proponents of SDM validly argue that patient autonomy is an essential aspect of engaging the patient in the management process, let alone a fundamental human right. If a patient has no part in the decision-making role, then how can they be committed to a course of action?

There is a lot of truth in this approach, but I think that it fails to appreciate the significant difference between knowledge and wisdom. Knowledge these days is so cheap that anyone with a $100 phone has access to nearly all the information (and misinformation!) in the world. It isn't necessary to have a medical degree to look up symptoms, signs, tests, treatments, side-effects and options. Plenty of websites and half an hour of research will answer most questions.

What patients need is not access to facts but rather access to insight. The danger with SDM is that it can easily devolve to "all care, no responsibility". "I provided the patient with the information – they can decide for themselves, and the consequences, of course, will then be theirs alone."

Proponents of SDM will say this isn't true shared decision making, and I fully agree. The danger however is that this is how the philosophy of SDM is being taken by those eager to avoid responsibility.

Rather than being an excuse to put the onus back on patients to make the final decision, SDM should be used as an opportunity to provide information and explore patients' understanding. At a deeper level, we explore not just what they know and are thinking but also the values that inform their thought process. When we understand them, then we can provide an interpretation for them of what they are looking or asking for.

In other words, if our education and accumulated knowledge really makes us experts, no realistic amount of time with a patient will empower them to the level that we have. We simply know too much, have too much practical knowledge, and above all too much perspective about the implications of the options.

On the other hand, no matter how well we know a patient, we never fully know the backstory of their lives, their values and their priorities. If we are fortunate enough to have been their GP for many years, we may have a pretty good idea, but assuming too much at any stage is fraught.

How then to balance these competing tensions? Dr Mary Jackson, an early partner in my practice, stated it succinctly and beautifully:

Patients pay the doctor to do the worrying for them.

An essential role for GPs is to make sure the patient leaves the room feeling better than when they came in. We may not be able to provide certainty of outcome ... and if we can, it may not be the outcome that they want ... but we can reassure them that we have the matter in hand and their interests at heart.

Of course every patient is different; has different values, education and cultural constructs. At any given moment, every patient's emotional capacity to deal with the certainty of a poor diagnosis, or the uncertainty of not having a diagnosis will vary. And every patient will have different interest and ability to absorb and digest information, then respond with a well thought out response. And the higher the stakes, the more likely a patient will react with an amygdala response rather than a cortical one.

This applies also to their families. Critical moments – a major illness, end of life care, shock revelations – can tear families apart because they revert to default settings and primal relationships.

This is not a call for paternalistic medicine. It is a call to never abandon the responsibility to be the person in the medical relationship who holds the power of both knowledge and wisdom, and therefore has the obligation to ensure that decisions made are genuinely in a patient's best interest.

When a patient is insistent on a clearly poor decision – one that is genuinely to their detriment – it isn't adequate to accept it as their choice. You have to commit yourself to find out why they are making that decision; to understand what are the drivers (emotional, physical, spiritual, financial) that lead them there, and then to challenge any incorrect assumptions.

A patient's decision doesn't have to be perfect, and it certainly doesn't have to be one we would make! But it does have to be reasonable – and in dubious cases we are usually much better placed than our patients to make that determination.

CHAPTER 34

Being Clever Isn't Clever

General Practice is overwhelming at first. Eventually it isn't.

At first everything is new and difficult. But with time, practice, study, repetition (and great supervisors) it gradually gets easier. What used to be cognitively and emotionally demanding becomes easier, then straightforward, then routine, then automatic.

Diagnoses that used to cause anxiety due to uncertainty are now elementary. So when a father brings in his daughter and describes a pearly little lump with a belly button in the middle, you can say molluscum contagiosum quicker than Dad can roll up her sleeve to show you.

Why shouldn't you? It's a marker of how knowledgeable and experienced you are. You're saving them time, moving on to the next thing they might want to talk about and perhaps saving a few minutes for the next patient who is waiting.

But I strongly advise you – whenever you immediately know what a problem is – not to say it!

Patients hate spot diagnoses.

To repeat a previous message – patients want you to show your clinical skill, but only after you've shown your level of care. If you make an instantaneous diagnosis, how carefully can you have actually assessed and considered what's going on? And if you haven't spent time thinking – then how could you possibly care?

The less familiar the patients are with the condition, the more you need to prove that you didn't just make up a silly diagnostic name to cover up your ignorance – molluscum contagiosum for example!

Show the patient (and the parent) that in your mental processing you have considered all the things that they have asked about – and even better, all the things they are thinking about but haven't mentioned. This is yet another reason to ask about their ideas, concerns and expectations.

Whilst this is obvious for problems that are physical and lend themselves to a visual spot diagnosis, it applies equally to psychological issues that also may be metaphorically diagnosed from the foot of the bed. A patient who has gone through a painful divorce after a messy separation may not accept that his tiredness is due to a "stress letdown reflex", even though you might sense it just by how he walks through the door.

You should also explain why your verdict is that their problem is psychological or physical – because the patient who thinks his issue is psychological needs proof it's physical; and a patient who thinks it's physical most definitely needs to be convinced that it is psychological.

An analogy I find useful is to explain that "If someone sticks an icepick 3 inches into your brain – you'll get a headache. If you sit with your neck at a 30-degree angle for 24 hours straight whilst working on your computer, you'll get a headache. If your cat dies, your partner leaves you, the tax office comes knocking and your car breaks down, you will get a headache. In each case the headache is real – but sometimes the headache is physical and in others psychological."

Using this analogy helps patients understand that psychological problems are no less real than physical ones – they are just different, and that you are not being dismissive of their concerns by fobbing it off as all in the head.

The patient needs to see, hear and sense you think your way through their problem, because that's the evidence that you care. You need to take the patient along that journey.

CHAPTER 35

Patients Or Paperwork

There are many things that registrars do better than their supervisors. Probably number one is clinical notes. In general, quality and quantity of a doctor's notes are inversely proportional to age.

Well do the MDOs say "Good notes, good defence; poor notes, poor defence; no notes, no defence."

We write our notes for only three people:

Ourselves – so we remember where we are up to in the diagnostic process and not embarrass ourselves by asking the same questions or ordering the same tests all over again; and where we are up to in the management process so that we don't retry treatments that have already failed.

Our colleagues – particularly in an era of group practice, so that others know what our thought process was if they need to step in during a diagnostic process or in the management phase of a chronic illness – such as where a patient is up to in their annual diabetic cycle of care.

The Judge – because she will want to know what happened in that consulting room when she has to decide whether our care was reasonable.

But writing up notes takes up about 25% of consultation time, and sometimes you need to compromise.

Sometimes you have to choose between comprehensive notes and a comprehensive consultation.

That's heretical in this era of medicolegal uncertainty, and I strongly suggest you debate this idea with senior doctors that you trust. In fact, it can well be argued that the exact opposite is true. The more complex a consultation, the more important detailed notes are. Yet perversely, a complex consultation leaves you less time to really think about your notes and write them up because of the need to move on to the next patient who has already been kept waiting longer due to the complexity of the previous patient!

This tension and the compromises it forces on us is rarely spoken of, but reflects the reality that time is the single biggest pressure in general practice.

In the months as I write this, our practice has trialled an AI scribe, rejected it and is now trying another. The hope is that these will relieve some of the physical, time and cognitive burden of note writing, though far from all. Every note that an AI engine writes must be carefully scrutinised. Things said and done will be missed; things not said may appear. No matter how accurate your software has been in the past, read every word it generates, every single time.

Reading may not be enough. I find it good practice to force myself to do one or two edits in every consultation note, just to ensure I am actually thinking about what I am reading. Our human tendency is to look for similarities. That means that in skimming the AI generated record, we will notice what matches up with the consultation, rather than what the software left out that we might have written ourselves. Don't outsource your thinking to an AI.

AI scribes are still nascent. The RACGP has declared that registrars should not use them in their first term of training, though I would urge you not to use them at all during the whole of your training period, even if your practice makes them available. Writing notes helps shape your thinking and formulate your plans. Writing brief yet comprehensive notes, accurate but not too wordy is a skill that takes practice. If you let the AI do it, you won't have a chance to become an expert yourself. When the time comes that you need it most – a practice that doesn't have AI, a home visit, a power failure, a really complex consultation – you will be least able to step back up.

What frightens me most is that if you rely on AI to write your notes, you won't be developing your own style. Rather than training the machine to write notes the way you want, it is likely you will adopt the structure, phrasing, conventions and style established by a non-medical programmer in Brisbane or Bangalore.

Apart from the three readers above, it is possible, as is slowly emerging, that our notes will also be written for the most important fourth person – the patient. Currently, in most practices, patients can only access their notes by formal request, and often this is done in conjunction with a consultation that explains what the notes mean. But there is a trend for doctors – especially geneticists and paediatricians, but slowly GPs also – to email their notes to the patient as a permanent record.

It makes sense – it's well established that patients remember only a small fraction of the information provided during a consultation.

But sending our raw notes to the patient poses its own problems, for the language and style that a doctor uses in writing notes for themselves and their colleagues is (and should be) quite different to that which one uses in giving an explanation to a patient. If we use medical jargon in our letters to patients, I am not sure how much clearer their understanding will be than from our verbal explanations. And if we only use lay-language in our notes, then we lose the precision, nuance and professionalism of our training.

The alternative is to write an intentionally drafted summary letter of our notes to our patients after each consultation, or at least the more significant ones. This idea has merit, but who is going to pay for the time involved in crafting a careful letter? Maybe – one day – that will be the most useful role for AI. I still doubt I will ever let a machine tell a patient what I said without reading and editing its choice of phrasing very carefully.

CHAPTER 36

School Days

There is a reason the medical course is long – six years "back in my day", perhaps five years now if you did undergraduate medicine, perhaps 8 years if you did postgrad. There's a massive amount to learn. At the time, the relevance of much material seemed highly doubtful.

But our teachers, and their teachers, developed this course for a reason. When answers are obvious, we forget how we got there. During our preclinical years, our clinical student days and then our early residency we filled our brains full of facts that initially was a jumble of data, and eventually synthesised into a coherent body of knowledge. Eventually it develops into insight and even wisdom.

When you start looking at moles, you go through a checklist of site, size, edge, colour, variation, bleeding, itch etc. Eventually you look at a mole, and you just know.

What applies to skin applies to most things. In your first year or two (or ten) of general practice, every presentation brings on a little panic attack. The joy of general practice is it consists of the patient who walks through the door, who may be bringing you the gift of talking about anything. That's also what makes it so terrifying.

But eventually you will have seen most things. Common things are common, and even rare things show up often enough that you won't feel overwhelmed. Still, every now and then – more in your early years, less later on, but always whilst you are a true GP – someone will come in and you will have no idea. Not just no idea about the diagnosis, but not even about where to begin testing, or examining, or taking a history. No idea at all.

When you don't know – go back to university.

It isn't necessary to reenrol at your alma mater. Just think about the problem, break it down, and roll back the years in reverse order.

Start by thinking about the clinical specialities. Is this problem likely to be medical, surgical or other? Which subspeciality?

- Medical: Addiction, Allergy, Cardiology, Dermatology, Endocrinology, Environmental medicine, Gastroenterology, Haematology, Immunology, Infectious disease, Neurology, Oncology, Pain medicine, Renal, Respiratory, Rheumatology, Occupational health, Pain medicine, Palliative care, Rehabilitation, Sexual health, Sports medicine, Toxicology.
- Surgical: Cardiothoracic, ENT, Head and Neck, Maxillofacial, Neurosurgical, Ophthalmological, Orthopaedic, Plastics and Reconstructive, Urology, Vascular.
- Age or Sex related – Andrology, Gynaecology, Obstetric, Fetal, Paediatric, Geriatric.
- Catch-all Other – Dental, Psychological, Psychiatric etc

If that doesn't help, go back one level and think about the clinical sciences. Don't try and solve the diagnosis, just think about the basic processes of disease. Is this a problem of

- Microbiology
- Biochemistry
- Genetics
- Pharmacology
- Nutrition

And if that doesn't help, go back to your preclinical years.

- Where is the problem – what's the anatomy?
- What isn't working – what's the physiology?
- Is this a medication effect – is this pharmacological?
- Is this psychological?

And if that doesn't work, then ask at the most basic level:

- Is this a question of structure or a question of function?

This is the epitome of slow thinking. Not relying on your instinct – your instinct has let you down. But trusting yourself that you know an awful lot – that's why they call you doctor – and that you can break this down by a process of inclusion and elimination.

The other helpful tool is to work through a checklist of pathological processes one by one. I'm not great at remembering mnemonics, but a helpful one is to worry that the VICTIM DIED IN PAIN:

VICTIM	**V**ascular	**I**nfective	**C**ongenital
	Traumatic	**I**atrogenic	**M**etabolic
DIED	**D**egenerative	**I**llicit drugs	**E**ndocrine
	Doctor's drugs		
IN	**I**nflammatory	**N**utritional	
PAIN	**P**sychological	**A**utoimmune	**I**diopathic
	Neoplastic		

Not knowing is half the fun of medicine! The reason maths is a prerequisite subject to enter the medical course is not because calculus is critical to being a good doctor, but because we have to be good at problem solving, and logically thinking our way through the riddles which we face, often thinking at several levels simultaneously.

Consider your day as a series of logic puzzles and you'll never feel like you're working!

CHAPTER 37

Wanting Answers

As far as backhanded compliments go, average is well above average. A restaurant that is "average" is probably below average – certainly not one that you would go back to. Average is boring, average is commonplace, average is no better than anyone else – just normal – and most of us want to be seen as a little bit special.

But when discussing health, normal is the gold standard. After all, our pathology results are nearly always based around the normal distribution curve, where average (median, mode, mean) are normal. We don't want to deviate from the normal – in that direction (or when it comes to the bell curve, in either direction) lies disease.

So when you tell a patient that their results are all normal, they are usually relieved. They shouldn't be.

Normal does not always mean ok.

Scenario 1.

Mrs Jones – good news. Your tests are all normal. We've checked your cholesterol, sugar and bone density. Everything is fine. Eat well, exercise, sleep well, see your dentist, do kind things for other people and I'll see you later in the year for your immunisation boosters.

Scenario 2.

Mrs Jones – the good news is that your tests are all normal. The bad news is that your tests are all normal. Your blood count is fine, your ferritin is fine. Kidney, liver, thyroid, sugar are all exactly where we would want them. Your ultrasound didn't show anything and the CT showed nothing to worry about. Everything is normal. But I still don't know why you are so profoundly tired, losing weight and have that pain in your abdomen.

If trying to exclude disease – normal is good. Screening tests for bowel cancer, human papilloma virus or diabetes are most pleasing when they come back without anything noteworthy. You don't want to be an interesting patient!

However, if doing tests to look for a diagnosis, normal is problematic. When we are hunting for the cause of a symptom, you want to know what's going on. A normal test might narrow the range of possibilities, but ultimately hasn't given you a clear answer.

When trying to make a diagnosis, normal is bad because you still don't know. Which means telling a patient that everything is normal isn't reassuring – it may actually increase their worry, because even the smart doctor has no idea. Which means it must be something occult, nasty, rare ... fatal.

There are also instances of inappropriately normal, e.g. a patient with serious infection but no fever, or a high fever without tachycardia, both of which suggest a patient much sicker than their normal signs suggest. This is particularly true in children and the elderly.

Be careful in reassuring a patient with normality until you can reassure them with an answer. At the very least, when doing diagnostic tests, be sure to tailend the explanation of normality with a very clear plan of what comes next. Are you going to do more tests? Refer to a specialist? Observe for a very clearly defined period of time with a fixed review at the end? Trial a medication? Under what circumstances – not just "if you're not feeling better" – should the patient come back?

Our role is not to do tests. Our role is to walk a journey with our patients and ultimately make them feel better. Normal test results don't make symptoms resolve, and certainly on their own don't make worry about symptoms go away.

CHAPTER 38

No-No

I think it's well established in medicine that we "always avoid always" and we "never say never". There is virtually no rule that doesn't have an exception, so giving any firm predictions is nigh on impossible. I recall one patient who had a miracle cure – with bone scans and PET scan showing multiple, untreatable bony metastases he was rejected from active care, went home, did nothing, and within a year all the metastases had disappeared.

Dr Peter Arnold, former Deputy President of the NSW Medical Board, taught me two other specific phrases to avoid. Arnold's dictum is to

Never say the word "just". Never use a phrase with "quick".

It might be "just" a routine procedure for you to perform or refer – but for a patient who has never had this before, it is a new, scary and perhaps terrifying event. Any surgery involves inconvenience, time, cost, pain, risk, complications and prognostic uncertainty. How is that ever "just" routine?

I might add my own interpretation. Why do we say "It's just a cold" or "It's just a virus" when somebody has an upper respiratory tract infection? We don't say "It's just pneumonia." We don't say "just a virus" when it's HIV – we don't even say it when somebody has herpes zoster, herpes simplex or Covid.

I think we say "just a virus" because we have no effective treatment for a cold. If we had a useful antiviral agent for URTIs, I am pretty certain that the standard phrasing would be something along the lines of "It's a significant viral infection – it's called rhinovirus. But do not be alarmed – I hold the power of cure, and I shall prescribe AntiVirulum that will resolve your symptoms within the week. I am the doctor – and I have spoken!"

For pneumonia, all manner of herpes, HIV and Covid we now have medications. We doctors have the capacity and authority to administer or withhold treatment. We have power over illness and patient. And power must be administered "justly" but not "just".

Similarly, we should never use the word "quick" as part of a phrase like "a quick check" or "quick exam".

Anything worth doing is worth doing appropriately. I don't know any GP who hasn't been caught by a patient who, as they reach for the door handle on the way out, asks "Can you just check this mole?" And you are now caught in a horrible bind. If you are to do this properly – get the patient adequately exposed, in good light, with a careful view and thinking about (and recording!) your findings and why you are deciding not to remove it ... you are reopening the consultation.

If you say "I'll just have a quick look" and that mole is a melanoma, or some other mole anywhere near that benign one turns into a melanoma in the next few years – what will be your defence? "I didn't have time to do a full examination"?

A quick check, look or examination is essentially no check, look or examination. The hard part of being a GP is being alert for pathology – cardiologists hear new murmurs every day; we have to really focus to stay tuned in to them. If you symbolically lay your stethoscope on a patient's chest without actually straining to hear a faint woosh, you have no chance of hearing a murmur. So why even try – you are not providing any true reassurance to yourself, and in most cases patients will be aware of how perfunctory your exam has been.

We all want to be helpful to our patients, and if they ask for "a quick xyz", we want to save them the time, expense, bother and wait of another appointment. It's too much to say that it's never appropriate to do a quick exam – but the occasions on which it is appropriate are few.

The same applies when the "quick" is driven by the doctor. If you are worried enough to want to do a cardiovascular or respiratory or abdominal or neurological exam, then superficial screening is probably not ever warranted. I appreciate that "a full neurological exam takes three days", but just moving the eyes in an H-pattern does not count as cranial nerve exam, and "olfactory nerve NAD" usually stands for Not Actually Done.

CHAPTER 39

Return To Sender

When I was a child, my GP had two pads on her desk. One was a script pad; the other a referral pad. The latter was just big enough to scribble down two sentences indicating the issue at hand, with three tick boxes at the top from which to choose:

☑ Opinion. In this case the patient would attend Melbourne's Collins St, Sydney's Macquarie St or the local equivalent in your town, where the specialist would conclude their consultation by stating "Well, Miss Brown, I've taken a history and examined you. I shall give the matter some thought and will write to Dr Jones shortly. That will be 3 guineas please."

Note that in this case the opinion belonged not to the patient but to the referring doctor! Certainly – and it's a good thing – that degree of patronizing is long gone. In a sense though, it hasn't. Radiologists almost never tell a patient what they think is going on – they defer that to the referring doctor, on the basis that the radiology findings can only be interpreted within the clinical context (which is largely true) but perhaps also gives them a reason not to need to speak to patients (which may be why they went into radiology in the first place!)

There is one other scenario where "opinion" has had a resurgence and that is the relatively new psychiatry 291 referral. In this case we ask the psychiatrist to conduct a single-visit assessment. They then provide us with a framework of management which we apply to manage the patient in the medium term with additional reviews if things don't evolve as needed. These are an incredible boon when done properly by both GP and psychiatrist as they expedite access, strengthen continuity of care and reduce the burden on specialist services. (They are also widely misused, a discussion for another day.)

☑ Immediate care. This was simply a request for a specific service by a specialist. "Dear Mr Smith – herewith Ms Brown with fever, vomiting and abdominal pain commencing at the umbilicus and now focused on the right lower quadrant. Please do the needful."

Immediate care is an easy referral. We are typically asking a surgeon to do something we aren't technically qualified to do, or perhaps a physician to sort out a specific symptom that eludes us. We are happy to resume full care of the patient once the matter is dealt with, and there is no need for ongoing review by the specialist beyond this episode of care.

☑ Continuing care. This might have been for a defined but lengthy period – "Dear paediatrician, please regularly see this child with congenital heart disease, intellectual disability, renal hypoplasia and intractable asthma. Please give me a call when the child turns 18 with your recommendations." It could also have been for a specific problem for a longer term – "Dear ophthalmologist – Mrs Brown has profound macular degeneration and diabetic eye disease. Please attend to these on a long-term basis – I'll look after the rest."

My understanding is that hospitals still use inter-departmental arrangements along these lines – please drop in and see this patient for a quick review; please help out with a specific issue so we can get on with our job; or please take over this patient, we have better uses for this bed.

In general practice however, the distinction has often disappeared. Some of that lies with specialists who are hungry for work and keen to keep reviewing patients who could easily be returned to sender. Other specialists have no idea of the skill set of GPs in general – or perhaps feel that their area of expertise is so refined that GPs simply can't keep up with latest essential developments, regardless of the knowledge of the specific GP who provided the referral.

But some of the issue rests with GPs who are less comfortable managing illnesses unless they feel they have complete mastery of the diagnosis and treatment. The problem is that you won't ever develop that mastery unless you start trying to do it. You aren't any good at cutting out ingrown toenails till you've done a dozen, and your first few wedge resections of pinnas – book in one hand, patient in the other – might be suboptimal. But unless you do them – you'll certainly never get better at them! And even if you have once treated Hepatitis C with antivirals – you may lose confidence if you've not done it for a couple of years.

Note that all of this is just as true for a surgical or medical registrar learning their craft – but they don't avoid the new for fear of the mistakes that they may make. They hunger for the opportunity to expand their skill set. They learn from their consultants. We can learn from both specialists and other GPs.

As a young GP, it's easy to start with a narrow range of practice, and as an old GP it's even easier to progressively shrink your scope. Instead, we need to proactively broaden our skills – medical, surgical and psychological – or we will indeed lose them. The letter G in GP stands for General – and it's important to remember that we need to maintain and continually develop that generalist, do almost everything, Jack-of-all-trades approach.

The trend to special interests in general practice was something that GPs once did after 10 to 15 years mastering the generalities, and was meant to rekindle passion within the profession, provide extra skills in a particular field whilst maintaining overall general care of a patient, their family and the community. I have deep concerns about "general practitioners" who focus on special and restricted interests as a way of avoiding needing to deal with the messiness of the breadth of general practice.

We also need to avoid the habit of referring off patients just because we don't like them or don't like the condition that they have. Dr Tim Diamond summarises this by stating that there are referrals to specialists and there are referrals away from general practice. It is important to know the difference, which you are doing and why. In other words:

When referring to a specialist – lend, don't send.

Sometimes patients need only short-term specialist input. But even if they need ongoing involvement from specialists for a particular illness, body part or treatment, we remain their primary care givers – primary in every sense of the word.

Don't let a specialist take over your patient's care – they rarely know the big picture of patient, past history, social situation, family illness and dynamics, local schools, shops and streets and especially how to deal with all the other aspects of the patient's health that have nothing to do with their area.

And please don't ask a specialist to take over your patient's care – they remain our responsibility until the day they move to another GP or die. We may not like them or be comfortable with them – but they are ours to care for, and we remain their GP no matter what.

CHAPTER 40

Autograph Hunter

Have you ever watched a magician at work? Not a conjurer, but someone who has truly mastered their job. The skill isn't that they do difficult things – it's that they make what they are doing look so easy that anyone could do it.

One of the greatest magicians I ever saw was a radiologist at the hospital where I did a term as medical registrar. In most hospitals a radiology round followed a familiar format. The registrar called out the case; the intern stumbled through the history; the radiologist pulled out the (hardcopy) films and interpreted the findings; the consultants provided the clinical verdict.

But this was different. Dr P, in his mid-80s, and already forcibly retired from a staff post under draconian hospital rules but allowed to return as a casual employee (five days a week for the past 10 years!) wasn't great at reading an ultrasound and didn't always know which end of a CT film was up.

But put a plain x-ray in his hand and he was a magician. The registrar would name the patient, the radiologist would put up the film, stare at it for a moment and then he would tell us the patient's history – what her presenting symptoms were, what the physical findings were and a whole lot of information about past history that the intern (shame-faced) had missed in his admission notes.

As someone who had spent 50 years with no radiological tools to hand other than plain and contrast x-ray, this particular consultant could read films like they were newspaper headlines.

A few months later, I started permanent work at my current clinic. There my local radiologist had an almost templated final line on nearly every x-ray report: "Further information might be gleaned from an ultrasound examination."

This wouldn't have been so bad, except virtually every ultrasound report concluded with the words "Further information might be gleaned from a CT examination."

MRI was not yet a thing, but many years later, on the very rare occasion I refer a patient to that radiologist, you can guess what nearly every CT report recommends.

Note that his plain-film reports don't recommend going straight to MRI – that would mean that the radiologist misses out on billing an ultrasound and CT first!

From these two experiences I have learned

The most important line on a radiology report is the signature.

Whilst radiology companies love to promote how up to date their scanners are and how modern their facilities are, the quality of a radiology service lies much more in the operator than the equipment. Chemical pathology and haematology are largely industrialised processes where the instrument determines the quality of the results. Very little interpretation is required. But radiology is highly operator and interpreter dependent.

True, radiology is probably the area of medicine most vulnerable to being replaced by artificial intelligence agents. Machine reading is rapidly reaching the stage where it can pick minor changes on a CT that are near invisible to the human eye – except perhaps Dr P. In turn this is going to lead to massive overdiagnosis which will bring us back to the need for a human filter of how significant each of these minor changes are. And in any event, the legal system will insist on someone signing off on the report so that someone is liable to be sued.

For now, histology and cytology are the two subspecialties in pathology where knowing who is reporting is as important as what is being reported. If you know your histopathologist, you know how readily she will upgrade a dubious melanocyte into melanoma-in-situ, or downgrade an early Bowen's disease into solar keratosis.

By extension, you need to learn the nuances of all your specialists. With time, you learn who to trust, what to trust, and when to trust them. I trust that you will find a cohort of specialists worthy of your referrals.

CHAPTER 41

Slow, Stop, Go

One of the first things that we learned in medical school was the role of the autonomic nervous system. Our primordial response to moments of stress is to activate the sympathetic nervous system and to respond with fight or flight.

In an ideal world, such primitive reactions have no place in our consultations. One of the hallmarks of being a professional is to remain in control of your emotions and to provide a detached, objective and considered response both to the problem and to the patient.

But inevitably there are consultations where things go badly. Perhaps it is a difficult patient – someone angry, upset, stressed by their life circumstances or by being kept waiting when they have somewhere to be. They might be under financial pressure, or suffering marital discord, or be miserable in their job, family and life.

Perhaps it is because the consultation itself is terribly emotionally charged. You might be breaking bad news; or needing to tell a patient something they don't want to hear.

It is even possible that the difficulty in the consultation lies within you. We are, after all, also human with human emotions, failings and stresses. When we are on top of our game we can either leave those personal feelings at the door, or at least recognise them, and in so doing control them enough for them not to have an impact on the consultation or patient. When we aren't at our best we might lay the impact of our burdens onto the patient.

Whatever the reason for the breakdown of a consultation, it is usually clear that something bad ... really bad ... is going on. The patient may raise their voice. You might respond in kind. The patient gets argumentative. You dig in your heels. The patient sits upright with an angry look in their eye. You feel threatened and uncomfortable and want the consultation to be over as quickly as possible.

At this point you can do one of three things. You can escalate the drama; yell back, demand the patient leave, push the panic button. You can walk out the door yourself and tell the practice manager to ban that patient. Or you can acquiesce and give the patient everything they asked for, reluctantly, with instructions that they are not to see you again.

For obvious reasons, all three of these are unsatisfactory solutions.

If you want to get the consultation over as quickly as possible – don't!

It's natural to want a bad situation to be over as quickly as possible. But the problem doesn't go away just because the patient leaves the room. Whether you are trying to provide great medical care, or are just concerned about avoiding a formal complaint to the practice or the medical board, the situation is not going to be better because the patient has gone. In fact, it is far more likely to get worse, because an incomplete consultation will fester in the patient's mind (and their subsequent conversational replays) without you there to defend yourself or to improve the outcome.

But there is a fourth option, at least before the consultation reaches an absolute point of no return.

When a consultation is going badly, stop the consultation and say, "This consultation is going badly."

What you are doing is trying to reset the consultation to the very beginning. A useful follow-up line is to say "I am not sure why we are disagreeing so strongly. Either I have failed to understand you properly, or I have not been clear in what I am trying to explain. Can we please try and work out where I am getting this wrong."

It's really important that you take primary responsibility for any misunderstanding that is going on. First – it truly is our job to make the consultation work. We are the professionals and that means taking responsibility for the flow and the outcome of the visit. It may not always be our fault when things go wrong, but more often than not, it actually is. The vast majority of consultations that go wrong do so because we haven't properly understood or addressed the patient's agenda. (Go back and read Chapter 1 again and again!)

But even if to an objective observer it is clear we have acted completely reasonably, and the patient is totally at fault – a rare enough occurrence – it is still our job to be the grownup in the room and accept the lion's share of responsibility. Turning the onus for the communication breakdown on ourselves forces the patient to agree with us. That in turn means that, even momentarily, we are on the same side and the push and pull of "I want my sleeping pill/antibiotic script/3 months off work certificate" is temporarily put on hold.

Stopping the consultation, particularly when you shoulder most of the blame, shows respect to the patient which will go a long way to reducing the tension. Obviously the earlier in the disagreement you do this, the less damage will have been done and the less entrenched the parties will be in their positions. But it does work even relatively late in the process.

In fact, this technique is still useful even if the consultation has deteriorated to a much greater degree. When you and a patient are bitterly disagreeing over everything, it can be helpful to simply say "I can see you are really angry." Well, how can the patient disagree with that? Which breaks the cycle of Yes/No; Black/White; I'm right/You're wrong.

It's much better if you never need to use this technique. But if you find a consultation is deteriorating and you are wishing the patient would leave the room as quickly as possible, you will find this a useful way of preventing a poor consultation degenerating into a poor review, a formal complaint, legal action or, most importantly, a patient who leaves dissatisfied that they did not receive the care they feel they deserve.

It should go without saying that none of the above applies if you are physically endangered. In that case, press the panic button, call for help or just get out of the room as quickly as you can.

CHAPTER 42

When Enough Is Enough

General practice is full of uncertainty. General practice is full of compromise. On behalf of the profession - sorry about that ... and live with it!

Living with the tension between competing demands isn't just a mindset; it's a skill that needs to be developed. It's very easy to fall into patterns of behaviour, not because they are correct but simply because it makes things easier if you aren't challenging yourself constantly to do a better job.

For some doctors that means resorting to perfection. The registrar who chases every minor pathology change (and there will be plenty – see Chapter 14) may tell herself that she is being careful, but in reality she is going to drive herself insane by refusing to admit that not every abnormality has an explicable cause.

For others, sanity is found in the plausible rather than the probable, or in the probable rather than the absolute. This registrar, having found a simple, reasonable explanation for a constellation of symptoms, doesn't look any further, because you can only hang a murderer once. But STIs for example, notoriously travel in packs. The young man who presents with dysuria will be pleased to learn that you found it was chlamydia and have treatment for it. He will be less pleased if he learns, 20 years later, that you didn't think about whether he might also have contracted syphilis.

Distinguishing between when good is good enough; and when it isn't, is vital. For many GPs, let alone registrars, it's the most challenging part of the job. We don't want to over-investigate. We don't want to under-investigate. We don't want to pathologise the normal, and we certainly don't want to dismiss the pathological.

Danish philosopher Soren Kierkegaard said that life must be lived forward but can only be understood backward. The retrospectoscope is well known to be the most accurate medical diagnostic instrument, but is most commonly wielded by those who weren't in the consulting room at the time of the presentation.

The first decision we have to make then is when to wait and see, when to keep looking with more tests, and when to pull out the script pad or scalpel and get on with doing something.

The mathematical formula for this is to multiply the square root of your concern by the floor value of the patient's anxiety level, divide by 85% of the rebatable cost of the test or procedure, raise the result to the positive predictive value of the court and then throw away the answer. Because unless the answer is obvious, in which case you wouldn't be angsting over what to do, there isn't going to be a right answer. There will however be several that are reasonable.

Wise King Solomon had a coin which he looked at to remind himself of his place. On one side it read "For you was the world created." On the other it read "You are nothing but dust and ashes." The circumstances dictated which side he looked at.

And so every GP needs a coin which on one side reads:

Perfect is the enemy of Good.

And on the other side.

Good is the enemy of Perfect.

What to do with the new patient who hasn't seen a doctor in years? He is visiting from interstate for two weeks before going home. Although he presented with a twisted knee, you providentially measure his blood pressure because it's a first visit and you're a good doctor. The sphygmo reads 187/102. You repeat it. Same result. After 10 minutes with the nurses – same result. What now?

You could do bloods and a urine test – if you think he would comply. And would you include lipids, for example, when you know that you won't be able to take long term responsibility for the result, and in the short term they don't really matter? You could ask him to come back in a day or a week to repeat the blood pressure – if you think that he will return and if you believe that everything is due to white-coat hypertension that will have disappeared at the next visit. You could arrange a 24-

hour BP monitor, although he doesn't fulfil the MBS criteria (his blood pressure is too high!) so he either pays for it privately or you take responsibility for cheating on the request slip. You could ask him to do home monitoring for two weeks which would involve him buying a machine he doesn't want and assumes he will follow up with someone, somewhere, sometime. You could ask him to see his own GP when he returns home, thoughtfully providing a letter, hoping for no adverse consequences in the interim. You could just start him on treatment that he potentially doesn't need. Or you could choose to do nothing – except see him again later in the week when he presents having had a stroke.

What you certainly will do is wish you'd never checked his blood pressure to begin with!

There isn't a right answer here. All of these choices seem reasonable to me, though you'll certainly find someone willing to criticise whichever choice you make. Younger doctors will tend to be more active more quickly in this scenario – older doctors would probably be more comfortable waiting a bit before starting treatment. (They, after all, know why manual sphygmomanometers go up to 300 mm Hg.)

Knowing that there often isn't a single right answer will help you distinguish between trying to get it exactly right and trying to get close enough. Get a sense for which matters most to the patient, to the illness and to yourself in which scenario.

CHAPTER 43

One Is Never Enough

Self-respect means doing the right thing even when nobody is watching.

The golfer who counts every stroke, even when playing a round solo is someone who is probably honest in every field of their life. Because the easiest person to lie to is yourself.

Just as spot diagnoses cheat a patient of the benefit of your knowledge and wisdom and experience and care, so too do spot diagnoses, or rapid diagnoses steal from you the opportunity to think.

Professor John Murtagh's diagnostic model – consider what is common, what is likely and what is serious – is powerful because it demands we contemplate what can go wrong. Without at least taking into consideration the worst-case scenario, you can't adequately plan for it.

Risk is a function of likelihood and severity.

So whenever you are presented with the gift of a problem by a patient, ensure that you think about multiple things you can do with that gift. Ideally, mention them to the patient so they know you have thought about them. But at the very least, articulate them to yourself (and put them in your notes). In other words:

No diagnosis is complete without a differential diagnosis.

Explicitly thinking of your differential diagnoses will save you from getting into trouble. The study of cognitive blindness is a burgeoning field of knowledge, but in a nutshell consists of identifying why we stop thinking too soon and either take first conclusions as correct or narrow our range of thoughts prematurely.

One technique – I don't use it but it has merit – is to list your differentials and assign a relative weight to each one. Thus you might assess that a patient with a chronic cough has a differential diagnosis list of – asthma (60%), COPD (30%), lung cancer (5%), other (5%). Spelling it out like this helps inform your treatment plan – if the lung cancer risk was 0.5%, you wouldn't start with a CT chest. If the risk was 15% you probably would, at 50% you certainly would. At 5%, it would be reasonable, depending on the patient's and your own degree of risk tolerance.

Even without allocating a percentage to each possibility, listing your differentials is useful because it puts in black on white just how broadly you have or haven't thought. Like telling a patient to write down their troubles (the list is rarely as long as they instinctively feel it is), writing down your differentials might show you that you haven't really considered that many possibilities, and that you need to think a bit deeper – or that the options are manifold and you need to start by prioritising.

My clinical notes are generally (abysmally) brief. But I do tell my registrars that if they ever find I wrote a lengthy entry to read it carefully. It means that I don't know what is going on, and my notes are a record not just of the patient's history, but of my thought process.

In complex cases, I will write my differentials list, and next to each one put the reasons both for and against. This sharpens my thinking, reminds me next time what I've already considered and/or rejected, provides a scaffold for the next doctor who might see the patient and demonstrates to the judge that I wasn't cavalier.

This habit is helpful for even simple cases, particularly early on. A teenager with a sore throat probably has a sore throat. Which means they probably have a viral sore throat. It's easy to check, reassure and dismiss. But once you've missed a couple of cases of glandular fever, you will, at first consciously, and later automatically, consider whether to feel for the spleen of every sore throat you see.

CHAPTER 44

Es Does It

An old joke. Einstein was once asked how Germany, perhaps the most culturally advanced country in Europe prior to World War Two, had given birth to the horrors of the Nazis and the Holocaust. He replied that when God created Germans, he endowed them with three characteristics – intelligence, kindness and Nazism. But because He wanted humans to have free will, He allowed each German to choose two of the three. Thus, said Einstein, if a person is a Nazi and intelligent, he cannot be kind. If a person is kind and a Nazi, he cannot be intelligent. And if a person is kind and intelligent ... he cannot be a Nazi!

Consider now, what are the hallmarks of a good consultation? It doesn't seem that difficult.

First – the consultation has to achieve what it set out to. There has to be progress in the patient's healthcare. Maybe not everything. But if she walks in with symptoms, she needs to walk out with a plan. If she walks in with test results, she needs to walk out with a diagnosis. In other words, the consultation needs to be effective.

Second – the consultation needs to be concluded within a reasonable period. General practice isn't an open cheque, and we need to ration our time – as painful and difficult as that is – with each patient. So every question needs to be asked with a purpose. Don't put the patient on the couch, examine one body part, sit the patient back in the chair, ask a few more questions, get them back on the couch, examine something else and repeat. Be sure the patient understands you, but once they do, don't explain something over and over again. In other words, the consultation needs to be efficient.

Finally – as we noted in Chapter 2 – the patient has to want to come back. It makes no difference how great the consultation is, if the patient doesn't think you have their best interests at heart, that in your eyes they are just a number to get back out the door. They need to know you are interested. They need to know you care. A consultation needs to be engaging.

These three aspects are all equally important -

A consultation must be the three Es - effective, efficient and engaging.

Of course those three properties are all in profound tension. It's very easy to do any one of them. It's less easy to do two simultaneously. But to achieve all the criteria – efficacy, efficiency and engagement – simultaneously is the great challenge.

When you spend time building rapport, then time working through the diagnostic process – you almost certainly won't have the patient efficiently out the door in 10 or 15 minutes. If you are briskly and brusquely efficient, practicing "strong medicine", being smart and safe in a reasonable time frame – then chances are the patient is going to feel cared for but not cared about. And if you practice what is disparagingly referred to as "have a chat" medicine, your patient will love you, you will be able to wind up the consult when you need to – but will you be any closer to a diagnosis, treatment or plan?

I know that there are few consultations where I feel I've hit the mark on all three.

To grow as a GP, reflect honestly after each consultation about in which domain you most fell short. It's easy to play to our strengths, but growth comes from working on our weaknesses.

CHAPTER 45

Exit Slowly

There's no such thing as work-life balance.

There is work-home balance, work-social balance, work-leisure balance, work-community balance – but not work-life balance. To use that phrase implies there is a dichotomy between those two things, on the one hand "work" and on the other hand "life" – whereas for most people work is a fundamental part of their life.

I see a lot of middle-aged men as patients. I spend my day telling half of them to work less, and the other half to work more. Work doesn't just provide an income – it also provides a sense of purpose, stimulation, validation, social connection, achievement, self-worth, communal contribution and a reason to get out of bed.

This is not to diminish the importance of leisure time. We need a break – each day, each week and several times a year. Hopefully during your evenings, weekends and holidays your head is less busy. A clear head is when you can actually reflect, with perspective, on what's going well and what could be better. Some of that might be active thinking but more often it is subliminal, unconscious processing. That's priceless in terms of becoming a better doctor and better person.

There is a thrill of anticipation as the time off approaches. The closer it gets, the more we think about the home-time or the weekend or the holiday, and that leaves less focus on the remaining work. You might even start to resent those last few hours or days before the break begins. I call this condition PHS - the pre-holiday shits.

Thus I implore you – keep your focus. That last patient needs you just as much as the one before and the one before that. He is just as entitled to your skill and care. Yet time and again we hear of doctors making mistakes just as they are glancing at the door. And so I urge you to:

Beware the last patient of the day; especially on a Friday; especially before a holiday.

Every snow-resort rescue crew tells tales of a skier who is tired at the end of a day or a holiday and is about to go home when they decide to go for one final run that frequently ends up at the medical clinic or hospital. The legs are tired, the focus is reduced, the joints are a bit achy. It only takes one poor turn to spiral into an unsteady run that ends in the trees.

I learned this lesson after making avoidable mistakes several times in the leadup to holidays. Perhaps that indicates that I should have taken holidays more often, but I think the key issue is the psychological let down just before the break, regardless of how often I take them.

On one occasion I did get it right, but someone else didn't. At 6:15pm on Friday 23rd December, just before the whole world shut down for Christmas, I got an email from our nurse. A 2-year-old walk-in new patient had presented in significant discomfort. "He is walking with legs apart, and upon looking can see his foreskin seems to be stuck down onto his sac. He is very uncomfortable and does not want us to touch. Unable to get urine spec as urethra blocked by position. Has not had wet nappy since 1300."

On exam his right testicle was swollen and was tender. Clearly torsion was possible, if not likely. I dashed off a letter, rang ED and went home.

I rang Mum the next morning and wasn't at all surprised to hear how busy the emergency department had been. I was much more surprised to hear that they took a quick look (see Chapter 38!) and had noted his swollen foreskin. They decided this was balanitis, told Mum the GP had overreacted and sent our young man home with antibiotics.

Grateful for the phone call – she was after all not our regular patient – she asked what she should do. I urged her to go back to hospital as I was quite certain this needed further assessment. And indeed, a few days into the New Year a hospital discharge summary arrived with an ultrasound report showing that on second presentation he was seen by a paediatric surgeon, admitted and an ultrasound had shown a torted testicular appendix. Fortunately, everything did resolve without complication.

I was lucky. The patient was lucky. And in my opinion, the first ED doctor was lucky.

The lessons are several. Every patient deserves your total focus and care, whether it is Monday 10am, Friday 6pm, or (if you do your own on-call) Sunday 4am. They deserve it for their welfare, and you deserve it because any patient can be the one that goes wrong. A momentary loss of concentration in the surgery is like a momentary loss of concentration on a freeway.

The other lesson is that specialists and hospital doctors aren't always right. If your gut says a patient needs prompt further assessment – by investigation, by specialist review or by hospital – then stick to your guns. Ask for it, ask again, and if the patient doesn't get it, ask for the name of the person who declines.

CHAPTER 46

Reasons And Excuses

It's common these days for businesses to have policies and signs that say "We have zero tolerance for aggression and bullying" (or violence or swearing or abusive behaviour).

It's an admirable message to send – not just to the public, but also to your staff and colleagues, that their safety is of critical, perhaps paramount, concern. But it isn't necessarily appropriate in general practice.

I'm not saying that staff should accept violence, or even aggressive, threatening, intimidating actions or language. I'm not saying that the customer is always right, or that patients can do no wrong.

But I am saying that

The illness is the illness.

If a patient has a necrotic wound, we might be put off by the smell, but we don't blame him for the offensive odour or refuse him treatment till the smell has gone. The stench is a byproduct of the illness, not something he can regulate.

If he has a gangrenous mental illness then his behaviour may be unacceptable, but consider carefully whether and how much he can control his actions.

Let's take a simple example and work backwards. If a patient is having a psychotic hallucinatory episode which resulted in him screaming into space in the waiting room, I don't think anyone would ban that patient from the clinic for life.

What if he yelled at a staff member during that episode? Yelled at another patient? Yelled at a young child?

What if he threw his keys across the room? Threw a chair?

What if he hit someone?

You can take a hard-line view that because he might do the last of these, we shouldn't accept the first. But where does that leave a patient with major psychiatric illness? Or you might take a lenient position that we will accept any behaviour that doesn't (maybe physically, maybe emotionally) harm anyone.

Just as a judge must determine whether a teenager's broken home is a mitigating factor in sentencing them after a car theft, we have to judge when to accept that a patient's illness is driving their behaviour rather than something innately immoral about them.

And just as the judge will, at age 20 or 30 or 40 say "Your desperately sad broken home is no longer an excuse for your behaviour now", or "We might forgive stealing a car, but not selling drugs to teenagers", you need to decide where a patient crosses your line of acceptable behaviour into misbehaviour, regardless of what may be causing it.

I don't believe there is a clear dividing line that applies in all cases, which is why I don't think that a blanket "We have a zero tolerance policy" is appropriate in reality, even if it is appropriate as a public sign.

Similarly, some practices have a sign saying "We do not prescribe drugs of addiction". Do they unfailingly stick to that rule? Or are they saying "We aren't interested in helping you"? When a drug-dependent patient is asking for drugs, we need to be careful to reject the request, not the patient. The enemy is the disease, not the patient suffering the disease.

The patient's illness will play out in multiple ways which can anger us, frustrate us or drive us to quitting medicine.

The patient with dementia who forgets to take his medications.

The patient with anxiety who can't organize his thoughts enough to provide a coherent history.

The disorganized patient who leaves asking for scripts till the last minute, then phones reception demanding they be written immediately as he is running out today.

The patient with poor health literacy who doesn't take his diabetes medications and whose glycaemic control goes from bad to worse.

The patient with OCD who asks for a letter to carry overseas explaining his medications, but rings multiple times wanting phrasing changed, the strength and dose of his vitamin tablets added, an explanation of why he is carrying repeats of some medications but not others.

The patient with a history of drug use and actively deteriorating mental illness who swears at reception.

The depressed patient who rejects every lifestyle suggestion that might make him feel just a little bit better.

My favourite line from Maimonides' physician's oath (see Chapter 50) is "May I never see in the patient anything other than a fellow creature in pain."

I have a copy of this oath on my consulting room wall. Before calling in certain heartsink patients (a horrible term – but we all use it) I re-read that line to ground myself.

The patient isn't responsible for his illness. But we are responsible for how we react to it.

CHAPTER 47

Lead And Follow

As an early career supervisor, I had the incredible privilege of learning from two giants. One was Dr Shane Fennessy, a supervisor par excellence whose untimely death led to the creation of a Supervisor of the Year award. From Shane I learned about how intimate the relationship between supervisor and registrar needs to be for a great learning experience.

The other was Dr Lindsay Quennell, an incredible teacher of teachers and mentor of mentors who taught me how to be an effective GP supervisor. One memorable exercise that Lindsay ran with us was to simply "draw a consultation". My art skills are worse than minimal, but the point was to do some form of schematic diagram.

When the time came to show our pictures, I was surprised. Some supervisors drew variations of the following:

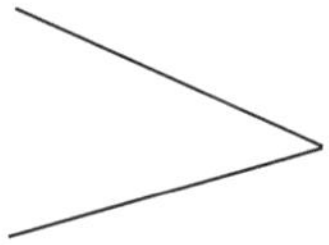

because a consultation starts incredibly broadly and narrows down as we refine with history, examination and questions.

Others drew

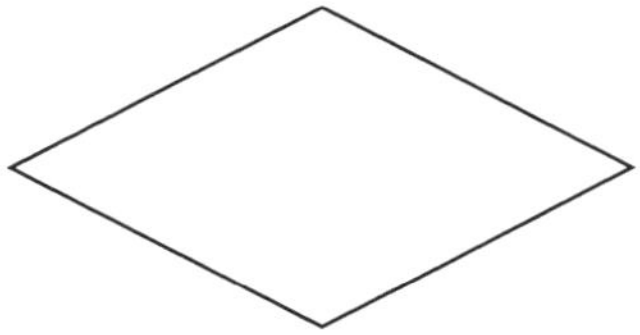

because a consultation begins with a single point – "How can I help you today?" and then broadens out as the history evolves before narrowing and refining down to a final conclusion.

Lindsay had developed his own model

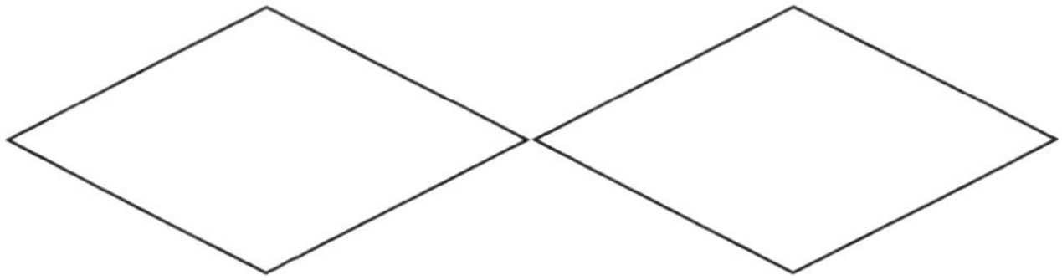

where the first diamond represents the history which belongs to the patient, and the second represents the examination and management phase which belongs to the clinician.

But of course, it was immediately clear to me that they were all wrong! For as soon as I understood the exercise, I had grabbed not one pen, but two, of contrasting colours and drew:

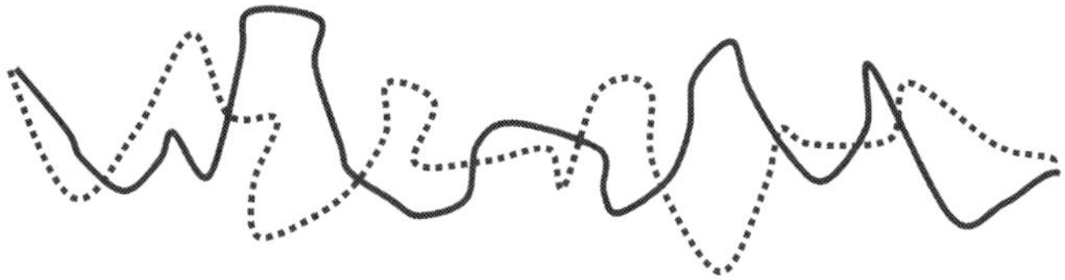

Where one line is the GP and the other is the patient. Because

A consultation is a dance.

Sometimes, particularly at first, the patient should lead. Later the GP takes on the primary role and the patient should follow. At times the two move in close synchrony, at other times there might be divergence and drift – which might be artistic, or might be damaging. But hopefully, like a Grade 5 school band, if we start at the same point and finish together it's pretty much been a success.

The dance metaphor is very helpful when a consultation seems to be meandering. A complex consultation rarely travels in a straight line. When the presentation is undifferentiated, when there are many possible diagnoses, investigations or treatments to consider, I might fall silent whilst thinking. I might pop out random questions probing for unlikely diagnoses, and those questions might seem totally irrelevant to a patient, while explaining the motivation underlying each question is just too time consuming and impractical.

A patient might then throw in a random bit of information which is incredibly helpful or totally irrelevant – they don't know and obviously they are trying to help you help them.

It's important in complex situations to pass the lead back and forth. "How can I help you?" and the patient is in charge of where the consultation goes. "Answer these specific questions" and you are. "Hop on the bed and be quiet while I examine you." But then you might return to the patient and say "What do you think is going on? What are you afraid is going on?" so that the driver of the consultation and the next steps belong to them. "Here is the plan" and once again you are leading.

As long as overall you are moving forward, the twists, turns and even double backs are what make complex general practice interesting! Enjoy the music. Enjoy the dance.

CHAPTER 48

On Being A Screen Star

There have been five major changes in medicine through my career.

The first three are now well entrenched. Smoking rates have plummeted from about 50% of patients to less than 15%. Medical records moved from cards to paper-based to computer-based. Practices have massively increased in size from 2-3 full time GPs to many clinics having 8-20 doctors, often part-time, and frequently working with in-house allied health and sometimes specialists.

The fourth change happened almost overnight during the Covid pandemic. Previously, many practices refused to provide any services to patients over the phone. If your child had a fever – they had to be brought in. If you needed a medical certificate lengthened, you needed to come in. If you wanted to know whether your pathology results were normal, you needed to come in (often only to be told that they weren't all back yet ... so make another appointment for tomorrow!)

The justification for this was that only by a face-to-face consultation could the doctor assess and examine you. Only face-to-face could the doctor know what the appropriate management was, and it was even (falsely) said that privacy laws meant that only face-to-face could the doctor be sure it was you she was giving the results to. Finally, the argument was actually put that if results were given over the phone, the patient may misunderstand and go and commit suicide!

Overnight that changed. Why? Because Medicare previously had a blanket ban on providing rebates for services over the phone. During the pandemic, telehealth suddenly was rebatable and practices could charge for telehealth services. Instantly all the objections to telehealth disappeared!

If you've not seen the film "All the President's Men" I highly recommend it. Among the iconic lines that come from that movie is the phrase "Follow the money." Money matters to most people, and doctors should be paid well for their work ... yet I cannot help but despair at the cynicism at play here.

In any event, telehealth – whether video or phone – is now here to stay and it brings its own benefits and challenges. Clearly it provides convenience and increases access. On the downside, the assessment of patients by telehealth is significantly limited. Obviously, there is no ability to examine a patient. But even beyond that, our communication with patients is very different in telehealth, especially telephone care where there are no visual cues at all.

From the GP's point of view, it's much harder to gauge a patient's mood, facial expression and body language when they are on a screen or not visible at all. Patients stiffen up on screen, their movements are restricted and there is an unnatural stare that makes interpretation much harder. Do they really understand the explanation you are giving? Have you sensed whether they've said everything they want to?

From a patient's perspective it is just as difficult. We doctors are also given over to staring at the screen rather than being more relaxed, and if we are typing at the same time, we aren't staring at the camera but just below it, which is very disconcerting for a patient who feels they are being looked past, not at.

When I was a registrar, we were frequently told to look at the patient, not down at the paper page scribbling our notes. Some of us even developed the skill of writing without looking – the manual equivalent of touch typing. When computerisation took hold, we were told that we must not stare at the screen ("the third person in the room") but keep looking at the patient.

Now with telehealth, particularly telephones, we don't look at the patient at all! If the point being made about looking at the patient is to capture their attention, just as they should hold ours, then how do we show them that we are focussed on them, when they can't see us?

Through trial and error I've learned that good telehealth requires even more energy than good face-to-face medicine! Though the problems by and large tend to be simpler, the inability to transmit information through expression and body language, the blunting of tone by the phone, means we have to be more enthusiastic, more energetic, more animated verbally than we would in a face-to-face consultation.

I'm not saying you should yell. But I do think that good telehealth requires additional thought and effort to ensure that you are getting your message across and checking that it actually has been received.

Regardless of its limitations, telehealth is here to stay. It can be a boon and it needs to be embraced as a useful tool.

Be enthusiastic about telehealth. Be enthusiastic during telehealth.

The principles I've discussed around telehealth – thinking carefully about the good and the bad; how it affects the consultation and the relationship; bending it to our needs, not diminishing our practice to suit its requirements – apply to all changes in medicine.

There will always be more. The next major shift, the introduction of artificial intelligence agents, is just starting. Beginning with digital scribes (and who knows what will follow), perhaps we finally will look at the patient much more. It remains to be seen if they want that! With increasing roles for AI in consulting, the future is exciting, frightening, dangerous and hopefully offers incredible improvements.

I won't be practicing long enough to see them all as a practitioner, but I look forward as a patient to smart doctors showing me how to harness the benefits without suffering from the deficits.

CHAPTER 49

To Err Is Human

I am going to make some assumptions. I assume you are smart – else you wouldn't have gotten into, let alone through, the medical course. I assume you care about people – else you wouldn't have chosen general practice. And I assume you want to be the best doctor you can – else you wouldn't be reading this book.

Registrars (indeed people) fall into two camps – the overconfident and the underconfident.

On the one hand, imposter system is incredibly common. Current wisdom is that this a self-imposed affliction primarily of women, but I have rarely met a good doctor of any gender who didn't harbour secret (or open) doubts about their true competence.

Indeed, I have only one recurring dream, even though I have been a doctor now for forty years. "They" come to me in the middle of the night and tell me that I didn't complete all the required assignments in final year medicine, I therefore didn't really pass, and all these years I have been practicing unqualified. I'm not really a doctor.

I am most certainly not the only doctor with those doubts.

On the other hand, doctors are quite like car drivers. By definition, fifty percent of drivers are below average (well, median at least). Yet if you ask nearly all drivers, they will rate themselves as "good" or "above average". Even those who confess to being below average (including me) are unlikely to rank themselves in the bottom quartile or quintile.

Yet again, by definition, somebody has to be there.

So also, with medical skills. I have never met a doctor who ranks themselves as below average, regardless of how strong the doubts about their own abilities are. How do we reconcile those two positions?

Mr Peter Grossberg, a general surgeon and excellent teacher, taught me in the 1980s that about 10% of open hernia operations fail and need redoing. Yet any surgeon would quote, hand on heart, and probably accurately, that at most 1-2% of their patients returned for repeat repair. Why? Because as a patient, if your operation failed, you are far more likely to go seek a different opinion and surgeon than return to the butcher who mucked it up first time round.

In other words, we see other people's mistakes more often and sooner than we see our own. So even though we fear that our knowledge and skills are substandard against some mysterious, external standard, compared to that GP down the road whose patients come to us for a second opinion, we are all Nobel Prize worthy.

Doctors, despite our reputation for closed ranks when it comes to medico-legal cases, are very ready to criticise and put down their colleagues. Yes, there are certainly some crap doctors out there, and certainly there are lots and lots of good doctors who sometimes make bad decisions. In fact we all do.

Depending on your personality style, you will probably travel through an arc of confidence as you enter general practice:

- I've survived 2-5 years in hospital. How hard can general practice be?
- Oh my God! In hospital I just kept telling patients to follow up with their GP ... and now I'm the GP ... and they're following up with me!
- I've got this – unless it's something I've never seen before – which is several times a day.
- General practice is just the gift of whatever issues the patient walking through the door is bringing me.

Somewhere in the middle of that range, you will start to feel confident in your own abilities, and in parallel, may feel smug or condescending about the mistakes that others make.

Then one day, you will be struck by hubris. You will make a mistake. You'll get an angry letter from a patient, or a request from a longstanding patient to transfer notes to another practice, or feedback from another GP in the clinic, or a comment from a patient's family that the specialist thought you had no idea what you were doing.

As painful as these moments will be, be grateful for them. Don't get defensive, don't shut down, don't lash out. Stop, pause, reflect. Though you won't feel thankful – you've been given a gift. This is a golden moment of growing.

More often than not, the learning will not be just about clinical matters, but also about the consultation and patient management aspects of general practice. Ask yourself not just how the mistake could have been avoided, but how can you better handle the situation post-mistake.

Remember that not all mistakes are avoidable. Sometimes the most reasonable path turns out to be the wrong one. General practice is full of incredible complexity, ambiguity and uncertainty. It simply isn't possible to always know what the right thing to do is without the benefit of hindsight, and it certainly isn't possible to always get it right when you are working with incomplete information and limited timeframes.

Underconfident doctors are dangerous because they are afraid to make any decision. Overconfident doctors are dangerous because they make decisions without proper consideration. Please,

Don't be confident till you've made mistakes.

It is possible to make the same mistake twice. But it's far more likely that you'll make lots of mistakes once. If you do that, and learn from them, you then will have reached the stage where confidence is justified.

Importantly, learn from other doctors' mistakes. Ask your supervisors and old time GPs for their war stories and "embarrassed to tell you" moments.

The working title of this book was The Other Man's Beard. It comes from a Yiddish proverb that "The wise man learns to shave on the other man's beard". Learn from the mistakes of others in preference to your own; learn from your own in preference to repeating them; and accept that some will happen throughout your career.

CHAPTER 50

Ask And You Shall Receive

There are many variations of and parallels to the Hippocratic Oath, and I recommend reading them to see just what multiple civilizations across space and time have in common as interpretations of the moral responsibilities of doctors, as well as the differences in phrasing and sometimes ideas.

One version well worth looking at is Maimonides' Physician's Oath, composed by Rabbi Moses Ben Maimon (known as Rambam for his initials) or Maimonides in Greek form. Maimonides was born in Cordova, Spain but primarily worked in Egypt and was famed not just for his medical knowledge and dedication to patients but also his mastery of both Jewish texts and classic Arabic and Greek works. His renown was so great that he acted as physician to both Richard the Lionheart and to Saladin – a Jewish doctor to leading figures in both the Christian and Muslim worlds at the time of the Crusades.

Amongst many pearls, one line in his version of the physician's oath stands out to me. "If doctors wiser than I wish to improve and instruct me, let me gratefully follow their guidance; for vast is the extent of our art."

In other words, though Maimonides may well have been able to claim the title of greatest doctor in the world in his time, he had the merit to remain humble and acknowledge just how incomplete his knowledge was. The fuller form of his physician's oath also includes reference to the importance of continuing medical education – well before this was mandated by medical regulators!

In a world where self-confidence is expected, humility is an ever-vanishing trait. Yet as doctors we will be bitten again and again when we show hubris. Humility is the prophylaxis against the long fall that sooner or later accompanies arrogance.

It's ok to not know. It's ok to say you don't know. In fact one of the easy aspects of general practice is that we rarely need to be the last line in the case of dilemma – we have the capacity to refer on nearly all of our diagnostic, management or relationship conundrums to other GPs or consultants.

But what if a patient wants a second opinion that you really feel they don't need? What if a patient has seen a specialist and wants another view after that?

There are two responses to this. The first is to tease out just why she wants a second opinion. Is it because she has no faith in the doctor's knowledge? Or that she didn't like his bedside manner? Or because she doesn't feel she can commit to a long-term care relationship with that physician? Or because she doesn't like what she was told and she hopes someone else will give her a diagnosis or prognosis that she will find more palatable?

Understanding the fundamental reason for a request for a second opinion will go a long way to helping you decide on whether it's appropriate and to whom the patient should be directed. Are we choosing someone with a different clinical skill set or a different personality and manner?

It's also worth respectfully asking the patient what she will do with the second opinion. If it's the same as the first one, what is the point of asking someone else? Would she follow up with the first specialist or the second? If the opinions vary – which will she believe? The one she wants to hear? Or maybe she would ask for a third opinion to settle the tie?!

At this point I find most patients withdraw their request. But if they persist, it's really important to agree to facilitate, even if you feel it is a waste of everybody's time and money to seek another opinion. Why? Because

A doctor who is offended by a request for a second opinion is someone whose primary opinion is not worth worrying about.

This applies equally to GPs who have given their own advice to a patient; a GP who has already referred to a specialist; and to specialists who have received a patient via referral.

In the latter case, if you as a GP ever get a letter from a specialist declining to facilitate a second opinion, or who tries to talk a patient out of it – delete him from your address book. That specialist has a badly inflated sense of his own skills and powers and is completely unaware of his ineffective bedside manner.

And in the first case mentioned above – if you ever get a request by a patient for a referral to a specialist as a second opinion to your own, always facilitate it. By all means ensure that it is not the result of the patient misunderstanding your advice. But don't argue and don't block. Your role as gate-keeper doesn't mean being a sentry-keeper. A graceful referral now may salvage a long-term relationship with a patient. A tug-of-war over a referral letter will alienate a patient, even if the specialist repeats verbatim what you already told the patient.

CHAPTER 51

World Weary Watch

The world is not divided into GPs and specialists. It is, according to world class cynic and world class GP Dr Steven Scully, divided into generalists and partialists.

Though we all graduate with a Bachelor of Medicine and Bachelor of Surgery (or variant thereof), we know that surgeons are a subgroup of doctors. Then came surgical specialties – vascular, ophthalmology, orthopaedics and general. But then general surgery split into abdominal and endocrine/breast. Then abdominal split into upper GI and lower GI. Then upper GI split into gastrooesophageal vs hepatobiliary.

Orthopods now concentrate on one or two joints. Indeed, in the USA, a friend had her surgery not by an orthopod, or a knee surgeon but by someone who only does soft-tissue knee surgery – ligament and tendon repairs but not knee replacements. Perhaps the next generation will subspecialise into left knee and right knee.

And they dare call general practice boring??!!

The issue for GPs is not that it's monotonous. It's that it is exhausting to always be alert. A cardiologist's ear is tuned into murmurs for she hears them every day. But we mostly see and hear normality. And if you've listened to the same patient's chest for 15 years, you don't really expect to hear anything new. But if you aren't really listening, really straining to hear – you won't detect the newly evolving aortic stenosis.

If you don't use it, you lose it. We don't look at enough retinas, and so when we do, we aren't sure what we are seeing. Doctors used to teach physios how to examine joints – now we get shown by them.

Fundamental skills are lost when not regularly practiced. Listen first, echo later! Examine breasts first, then do the US. PR and PV exams are now virtually gone. Sigmoidoscopy really is gone despite my surgical professor's dictum that no abdominal exam is complete without performing one.

If you don't look for pathology, you won't find it! Not just the theatrical motions of laying scope on chest, but actively listening to the heart as we would actively listen to a patient. We see and hear what we expect to see and hear. Unless you are searching for pathology – you won't find it.

It's not that general practice is boring. It's that it lulls you into a false sense of serenity.

And once it does – watch out.

One of the most memorable registrars I ever had almost didn't even get interviewed. She did her intern year, then took a year off to have a baby. She did second year – then took another year off for her second baby, and then wanted to start GP training. With so little continuity or intensity of experience in her hospital years, I thought she was very underprepared for general practice. But we received few applications that year, so I agreed to see her.

Not only was I blown away by her enthusiasm, but when she started work, I was astounded at her sixth sense for finding pathology. She introduced me to the phrase "shit-magnet" for the amount of pathology that came her way, but it wasn't that sicker people presented to her. It's that, without being paranoid, she was always alert to the possibility of finding pathology even though the presentation could be easily downplayed.

As final-year medical students we did a rotation in community health. The professor of general practice presented a case of a middle-aged woman with tiredness and an abnormal FBE. He asked for some differentials and one student – a high-powered physician-in-the-making – began by proposing acute lymphocytic leukemia. The professor looked down with disdain and said "I've been a doctor for forty years. Do you know how many cases of ALL I've diagnosed? None!"

To which a voice from the back of the room called out "Yes – but how many have you missed?"

CHAPTER 52

The Sum And The Parts

Very early on in your training – or lived experience – as a GP, you will be taught to "get the list" – that is, to have the patient specify all the problems they want addressed at the consultation so that you aren't blindsided at the end of the visit with a "Could you please check this mole", or worse "Actually what I really wanted to talk about was these pains in the chest that come on every night".

There is of course validity in asking the patient to provide "the list". In theory at least it means that you and the patient know what the issues are, and you can agree on priorities, and how much can be practically dealt with in the time available.

It usually also clarifies for the patient that their expectations are unrealistic when they keep raising additional issues, and then you repeat back to them what they want to address. My personal record, after repeatedly nodding and asking "and is there anything else?" was a new patient who came in with 14 separate problems!

It's terribly frustrating when a patient just keeps bringing up new problems every time you address the previous one, so settling on a list at the beginning should in theory restrict the consultation to what was agreed on at the start.

In chapters 5 and 31 we've already mentioned the concept of "ticket of entry" – a patient presenting with a minor problem as a way of checking out the doctor (even if well known to them) before they feel comfortable to talk about what is really bothering them – the rash, the discharge, the domestic abuse, the erectile dysfunction.

When we pressure a patient to put everything on the table initially, we shame them into not being comfortable to bring it up later. Perhaps the best compromise is to establish the list at the beginning but still end the consultation with "Is there anything else?" and then – unless life threatening – book the next appointment then and there.

There is a more subtle reason to get out the list, and that is to integrate what a patient might perceive as multiple problems into a single grand unified issue.

Often registrars deal with the issues on the list sequentially. They address the first problem, take a history, perform an examination, establish a diagnosis, write a script and develop a management plan. Next problem. Repeat.

This is neither time efficient, nor good medicine. It completely ignores one of the fundamental principles of science, Ockham's razor – that whenever multiple phenomena are observed, it is better to find a single explanation for all of them than a series of individual answers.

In other words

A good consultation may be a short case or a long case, but never a series of short cases.

Lest I seem to be lecturing you about your shortcomings, let me assure you I still make this elementary mistake often enough. A straightforward example from last week, when a patient came in for a repeat of her long-term anti-hypertensives. Which I printed before routinely checking her always well controlled blood pressure. Which was high. Necessitating a change in her BP medication. Which I printed. Then she mentioned her troublesome knee. For which she had been taking lots of anti-inflammatories. Which made me rethink the need for upping her BP medication. So I cancelled that new script and rewrote the old one. Then thought about her use of diclofenac. And asked about her abdomen. Which was tender. Which needed examination before deciding to prescribe a short course of proton pump inhibitor. Which meant at least mentioning the risk of osteoporosis given her strong family history. Which opened up a whole new consultation.

I hope you are squirming at how messy this consult was as much as I am when I write it all out. When you approach a consultation as a series of unrelated matters, your thinking becomes focussed on the micro instead of the big picture. Your history, examination and management will tend to the partial instead of the holistic. This will not benefit, but may certainly disadvantage, the patient.

It's also really dissatisfying for you. A series of short cases on the same patient will feel like 6-minute medicine even if you've spent 20 minutes with the patient – because it really is! If you deal with multiple problems in isolation, then it makes little difference whether it is one patient with three problems taking fifteen minutes, or three patients each with one problem taking five minutes.

What's off-putting about a patient asking you to throw in a script at the end of a consult is that every repeat script is actually a problem – a BP to be checked , an asthmatic chest to be reviewed, an antidepressant to perhaps deprescribe or a hypoglycaemic to step up and down. But then the dietary discussion around BP overlaps with the exercise discussion around diabetes control which leads into the social prescribing management of depression.

The fun of a jigsaw puzzle isn't putting two random pieces together – it's inserting the final piece that completes the picture. Treating any one problem in isolation is frustrating. It's only when you synthesise the entire consultation into a unified whole that you will be truly satisfied.

CHAPTER 53

Right Person, Right Tool

If GPs deal with everything and specialists have a narrow scope of practice, why are general practice appointments generally shorter than those of specialists? Sensibly, given we deal with multiple issues and multiple systems, and very often at the same time – our appointments should be considerably longer.

Think about this – how long are initial consultations at your clinic – that is, the first appointment for a new patient? In nearly all practices the answer is half an hour – double a standard 15 min appointment. In some clinics that run 10 min appointments, it might be either 20 or 30 minutes.

How long are initial specialist appointments? Depending on the specialist and the speciality, they typically vary from 30 to 60 minutes.

Why the difference? At an initial appointment, we always take a full background history – including family, occupational, smoking, alcohol and drug use, past history, allergies and medications.

It's clear that many specialists don't!

We take a thorough history of the presenting issues. There might be only one, but very often there are multiple problems all laid on the table at the same time, and just sorting the symptoms into piles that make up a problem list can be time consuming in itself. Most specialists – certainly surgeons, and often physicians – are dealing with a single, clearly identified problem which (if the patient has a good GP!) has been well defined and worked up by the referring doctor. Of course sometimes there are diagnostic dilemmas, but very often the path forward is clear.

And, one hopes, the physical examination by a GP and specialist is identical.

Why then are specialist appointments so much longer?

Specialists cut with a knife. GPs peel back layers.

The intent of a specialist consultation is much more specific. See problem. Label problem. Fix problem. Move on.

A GP's work is never finished. We meet a patient, not with the intent of curing her, but with the intent of building a 20, 30, 40-year relationship with her. We will travel the journey – dealing with acute illness, chronic disease and preventative health matters. We will see her on her own and with her family. We will be the person she comes to when she doesn't know who to turn to.

Over time – if you really do see a patient regularly – you will know her as well as her closest family and friends do. Perhaps even more so, because she may tell you things she's never told anyone else. Whether revealing childhood sexual abuse, or her deepest fears about breast cancer, we can get inside her mind in a way no one else can.

But that cannot happen in a single visit, no matter how much time we spend with her. That degree of trust, empathy and relationship can only develop over time. Regular contact is more important than a single blast.

So our appointment book and our appointment structures are designed to do things gradually and steadily. This serves us well most of the time, though fails us when a patient really does need an extraordinarily long consultation (by general practice standards) to work through a matter. For weekly hour-long counselling like a psychologist, or a super-long appointment to do a full top-to-toe neurological exam, our regular consultation lengths don't work particularly well.

You can deal with that in two ways. One is to just book a super long appointment, which is fine enough, though often difficult in practical terms if your book is full and your days are busy. And of course Medicare rebates on a per minute basis are less than 75% for a (prolonged) Level D or (extended) Level E consult, compared to a (standard) Level B.

The other way is to break a consultation into multiple parts, using the initial visit of a new complex episode to map out a way forward, and subsequent visits to explore. We need not be ashamed if we have taken a deep history to defer the examination to another day, then review test results a week later, then ask the patient to return yet again for a referral or care plan.

We can trial a medication, see her in a fortnight, titrate the dose, review once more, add another drug, and review again. We exclude life threatening physical illness, then explore if there is an underlying mental health cause, then systematically work our way through the long list of differentials in order of severity or order of likelihood.

Specialists are in a rush and want to do it all in one hit, then and there. We are just as busy – but we need to be patient with our patients. We don't have enough time to be in a hurry.

CHAPTER 54

Start In The Middle

I've often had to accompany patients through a prolonged episode of illness – recovering from a major stroke or the profound grief from loss of several members of a family simultaneously. When the time comes for them to return to some form of normal life, the question arises of timing for return to work.

Often the plan is to return part-time, and this makes sense. Work is physically and mentally taxing and being match-fit takes time and exposure. To go from 0 to 100 after a long absence is asking too much.

When I talk to patients about this, I usually surprise them by strongly suggesting

After a prolonged absence, return to work on a Friday.

At first blush this doesn't seem to make sense. We start things at the very beginning. Surely recommencing work should begin at the start of the week, on a Monday.

My argument is that on the first day back in the office, very little work will be done. Often the patient dreads what is going to happen. The unknown of whether they can even still do their job. The uncomfortable first chat – everyone coming up to you, asking how you are, giving condolences or sympathies. There will be a mountain of emails to read, phone calls to return, meetings to set up and prepare for. For someone who hasn't been at work for weeks or months, it's all way too much. And if that is Monday, then Tuesday and Wednesday won't be very different, and the respite of the weekend is so very far away.

But going back to work on a Friday changes the scenario enormously. Nobody expects anyone to do a week's work beginning on a Friday. Instead of ducking everybody, it's a chance to let people come up and make any awkward comments that they choose. You get to hit delete on hundreds of irrelevant emails. You plan what you will do the following week – but you don't have to start doing any of it. And then, perhaps soon after lunch, you pick up your bag and go home. Nobody will say anything and no one will mind. Your weekend has begun.

All firsts are hard. If your week begins on a Monday, your first week back at work is five days long. If your week begins on a Friday, your first week back is just a single day. By Monday, your colleagues, having already done the necessary, awkward social niceties, will have moved on with their personal and work life, and reduced the pressure on yours. You don't have to spend the weekend before the first day anxious about how you will cope returning to work – you've already done it!

This notion of starting in the middle rather than at the notional beginning is a very helpful tool for us too. I often prefer to drop into work (or dial in remotely) over the last weekend of a holiday just to get a sense of what lies ahead. Reception and nursing staff always kindly protect us whilst we are away, by letting patients, specialists and lawyers know we are on leave, and that we will call them back when we return. "Oh – that'll be 9:00 am on Monday, March nth". Not much work will be done that day as dozens of patients ring wanting to know why they haven't been called back by 10am!

Coming back a day early for a bit of paperwork cleanup might seem like an awful waste of a final day of holidays, but in fact often makes for a much calmer return to work, rather than the chaos of a mad first day, by the end of which all feeling of holiday relaxation has gone.

Forestalling anticipatory stress is why I sometimes sneak a surprise onto my first-term registrars. We typically spend two full days in orientation at the beginning of the first week, with the registrars sitting in watching me consult so that they get a sense of how a visit works, how to use the software and how to bill.

Registrars with an activist learning style want to get that over and done with so they can start consulting themselves. But those who are "reflectors" never feel fully prepared to actually start. I've often noticed amongst that cohort that late on the Tuesday their anxiety levels visibly build as the Wednesday morning starting gun looms. To bypass that, we often ask them to see one patient late on the Tuesday afternoon, with very little warning. Invariably it isn't as scary as they expected, and they sleep all the better that night for their first general practice consultation is now behind them, not an unknown dread to be faced the next morning.

CHAPTER 55

First This, Then That

Whilst we rapidly approach a cashless society, we aren't quite there yet. So here is a little thought experiment. Describe to someone who has never had to do it, exactly the steps for taking cash out of an ATM.

You go to the ATM. You put in your card. You enter your PIN. You tell it that you want to withdraw cash. You enter from which account. You enter how much. You take your cash. You take your card.

Actually, that's wrong! That was indeed the order when ATMs were first introduced in the 1970s. But then banks noted a common error. Customers would take their cash, turn around and walk off. The machine would spit out their card, but it was too late – the customer had already left.

The remedy was simple. The last two steps were reversed. The machine would first push out the card, and then the cash came out. Problem solved – people took their card back because it popped out while they were still focussed. And nobody who visits an ATM forgets to take their cash, whether it comes out first or last. That's the whole point of visiting an ATM.

Chapter 41 emphasised the difference between striving for good and striving for perfection. Doctors tend to be perfectionists, and perfectionists can obsess over minor points of difference. Usually it doesn't matter much.

Nonetheless, if there are two ways of ordering a process, one is probably ever so slightly better than the other. It might not make much difference, and it certainly won't be worth redoing just so you can reverse what you've done should you catch yourself "in error" doing it in the suboptimal order. But repeatedly doing things in the right order means you'll develop habits that will help, even if just incrementally.

Thus I've learned a lesson:

Always recap the dipstick bottle before opening the urine jar.

When patients brought me a yellow-top, my aim was to do a full ward test. So I'd open the jar, open the dipstick bottle, shake out a chemical strip, pop it in the urine and whilst waiting for it to cook, I would recap the tube with the dipsticks.

Being both clumsy and a slow learner, it took me a couple of minor disasters to change my order. More than once, as I tipped the dipstick bottle to shake loose a strip, the whole contents would come sliding out, scattering over sink and floor, and more than one strip – sometimes the whole jar – landing in the open pot of urine. And sometimes spilling the contents of that container everywhere as well!

Brighter minds would have realised sooner than me that the fix is simple, and the nett difference in time is less than three seconds. I now take the dipstick jar, take or shake out one strip, recap the jar, and only then open the urine jar. No more risk of dipstick disaster!

It's not a lifechanging advancement in healthcare or running a practice. But if I can avoid wasting $60 of chemical strips, cleaning up a urine mess and being embarrassed in front of a patient – it's a good use of literally a couple of seconds.

There are plenty of other times when the order in which we do things matters just a little, but that little might as well be to your benefit.

My fiancée and I chose to honour the tradition of not seeing each other for the week before our wedding. (I highly recommend this – it makes the moment of meeting at the ceremony very special.) During that week I resolved to remove the sebaceous cyst on my scalp that she had never liked, and which was more obvious following my pre-wedding haircut.

So I asked a friendly surgeon if he would remove it. Being a proper surgical type, he asked me to meet him in theatre at the end of his list. He scrubbed, gloved, put some local into the scalp, which of course stung quite a bit – and started cutting. I yelled. The local hadn't had time to work. His response was to grab a syringe and head toward me with the intention of adding injury to injury. Clearly he had no time to waste – his favour to me was consuming valuable lunch time!

I stated the obvious – that he needed to wait for the local to kick in. He replied, "Some people just need more". I pointed out that local anaesthetic needs a finite amount of time to be effective. By the time we finished our 60-second debate, and he retested the field, the anaesthesia had taken effect.

So my habit is to reverse the order. With clean hands and no touch technique, put in some local and do the presurgical scrub. By the time I've washed, dried and gloved, nearly every patient reports complete anaesthesia at the site of injection. No waiting around, no awkward silence while the local takes effect.

You can find lots of opportunity to micro-optimise your day. I do three-monthly diabetic visits, asking patients to take their shoes off for a weight check twice a year. Since they are already deshod, I also ask them to take off their socks to check pedal pulses and sensation. On the alternate visits, they leave all their footwear on, and I save one or two minutes per consult.

Similarly, I don't print out my path form while the patient is staring at me. Or rather I do so at a time when the patient is looking at me but not able to do anything else – whilst the automated BP cuff is checking their BP. During those 45 seconds, there used to be a pause – I had nothing to say till the BP check was complete, and the patient wasn't allowed to talk, as it disturbs the sphygmomanometer's readings. So, very simply, I now print off the next visit's pathology form in exactly the time it takes for the BP machine to do its job. The patient can see that I'm busy, and I feel that I've used that time productively.

Once this becomes routine, you'll notice micro-frustrations forced upon you by others. For some strange reason, both the leading medical software companies record blood pressure in the order sitting, standing, lying. But if you are checking postural BP change, you should do lying before standing. It makes no sense for the medical notes to record them in the opposite order.

Simple changes of sequence, once ingrained as habit, make a big difference to the safety, speed or efficacy of your workflow. Think about the order in which you do everything that you do.

CHAPTER 56

Two Ears, One Mouth

I think it was my anatomy lecturer Professor Wilfred Brookes who taught "Revision is learning for the first time." Certainly repetition is a central part of internalising information and habits. So let me repeat something we've discussed earlier on – the importance of listening.

An adage says that we have two ears and one mouth because we should listen twice as much as we speak. That is certainly true in the medical field, particularly early in a consultation. Until you know what the patient has to say (their facts), and how they are saying it (their emotions) and why they are saying it (their motivations), you can have no idea what you are responding to, let alone the best way to do it.

We listen to patients for the superficial layer of communication called speech. We watch them for the deeper level called body language. We go a layer yet deeper when we ask ourselves "What didn't the patient say?"

A basic example is the patient who dodges the question "How much alcohol do you drink?" with the answer "Socially". Socially depends very much on your social circles! As a medical student my main psychiatry assignment was on a council-worker with Wernicke-Korsakoff syndrome, who had alcoholic brain damage from drinking 15 "long-necks" (750ml beer bottles) per day. But he thought he was a social drinker, because in his crowd, many of his mates drank 20 per day. (Just imagine drinking 12-15 litres of water per day, let alone beer!)

When a patient gives a vague response, they are usually making a choice to not say something. By now you certainly know when a patient says "social drinking" to ask how many? And on weekends? And at parties?

A deeper example of listening to what the patient didn't say is the late-30s woman who presented with vague symptoms of tiredness and headaches. She spoke of her stressful job and overbearing manager. She wondered if her difficult menstrual cycle meant she was anaemic. She mentioned her poor sleep patterns and her efforts with diet and exercise. But the more I listened to what in her life was bothering her, the more I realised what she wasn't speaking about. She made no mention of her personal life.

At that point, it wasn't too difficult to ask a few questions about her relationships – or rather their absence. Which then led to the question of her ticking biological clock. I don't think there was any way she would have raised this issue – because I don't think she even realised how much it was weighing on her until we named it – but her impending childlessness was, as it transpired, the primary cause of her depression and thus her tiredness, and was making her far more unwell than she realised.

When doctors speak, it is **our** words that fill the room, not the patients'.

When doctors speak, we are planning what we will say next, not thinking about the meaning of what the patient said.

When we speak, we are thinking about the accuracy of our phrasing, not the significance of the patient's unspoken thoughts, or unrecognised feelings.

When we speak, we rob the patient of the chance to be understood.

The more a patient talks, the less they'll feel you didn't listen.

And most importantly -

The more a patient talks, the more you'll hear what they don't say.

If you must speak – and of course we must! – how we do it is just as important. I must often remind myself that, to my mother's disappointment, I became a doctor not a lawyer. We aren't there to cross examine patients with a series of rapid-fire questions in an interrogation, looking for irregularities in the story that we can exploit to make the patient feel belittled! If I find a patient contradicting themselves, I point that out as a matter of my own failure to understand rather than their inconsistencies.

Dr Peter Tribe, whom we met in Chapter 7, has a wonderful way of taking a history. He seems to never ask a question at all. He just chats away with the patient as he meanders down the corridor, seemingly never in a hurry. He reflects on their last consultation or their family or the football, and yet somehow that leads to the patient blurting out all the symptoms of their indigestion which is actually cardiac pain, or their marital woes and subsequent depression.

It's almost magical to behold and I wish I could emulate it. At the very least I have learned that gathering facts is the most superficial component of history taking – listening to what is and isn't being said, how it's being said and why it's being said in that way is what really unpacks the layers of meaning behind why the patient has come.

CHAPTER 57

The Paradox Of Choice

"So Mr Brown – your blood pressure has been up the last few times we've checked it, and your 24-hour blood pressure monitor confirms you have high blood pressure. I think it's time we started medication."

"OK Doc – you're the boss. What are you going to give me?"

And now silence. What will you answer? Of course there are guidelines. Though they do keep changing, so if that's what you rely upon, you'd better double check. That decade it was diuretics first, next decade it was beta-blockers. Calcium channel blockers were great, then came ACEIs and ARBs, and then a shift back to alpha-blockers, at least as second line treatment. And now the circle completes with spironolactone again in fashion.

But you'd better be right because you know that as soon as you name a drug or a class, the patient is going to ask "Is that the best thing for blood pressure?"

Well – is it? You know that whatever you prescribe will probably work, but not definitely. Will probably have side-effects, but not definitely. Might be tolerated, or might not. How are you going to defend yourself when the patient comes back complaining of nocturia or nightmares or leg swelling or a niggling cough? Why did you pick something that you knew had such side-effects?

By being honest with the patient and yourself.

If there are many treatments for a disease, none of them are any good.

That doesn't mean they are all useless! It simply means that if one was exceptionally better than the others, market forces and clinical demand would drive the inferior products to extinction.

The fact that there are so many anti-hypertensives, diabetes medications, anti-depressants etc, is a function and marker of variation in statistical efficacy, individual responses, drug and disease interactions, tolerability of side-effects, cost, convenience and compliance and a myriad of other factors.

We grow up as doctors developing prescribing patterns and habits, and it's hard to shake those when we've prescribed the same medication for years, having seen newer, "better" drugs come along with great hype, only to be quietly withdrawn a year or five later due to newly appreciated side-effects. Far better to stick with what we know works pretty well, than potentially harm our patients by chasing the elusive perfect drug.

The burgeoning field of pharmacogenomics is perhaps going to be the great game-changer of medicine for the generation reading this book. Personalised medicine, if it lives up to the promise, will help guide the exact best-fit treatment in a way that I never had the chance to experience. For us it has been "suck it and see", with patients our willing, if unknowing, guinea pigs.

What applies to medications also applies to plenty of other choices and decisions that we make. It always entertains me when I recommend a patient go see a specialist and they ask, "Is he any good?" My standard response is "Oh ... did you want somebody **good**?!? Sorry ... I misunderstood. Of course, no, I'll send you to somebody else."

But how do we know that the specialists we choose are the right choice? Some will have been your teachers at university or your consultants in your hospital years. Later it will be your classmates or fellow residents who have now completed their training and are in private practice. Some will be the recommendations of the GPs who've been in your practice and suburb longer than you.

Eventually you'll develop your own referral pattern based on the letters you get, and the feedback patients give you. Truthfully, you'll never do a randomised controlled trial of which orthopod has better twenty-year outcomes in hip replacements, even though that's what you need in order to provide a recommendation about which surgeon actually is "the best".

We do the same thing for which we judge our patients. We often see the results of bad medical practice at other clinics, yet patients swear by those GPs. We know they are confusing bedside manner for clinical competence. Yet by relying on soft endpoints rather than hard data, we are building our prescribing and referring database on exactly the same sort of anecdote rather than evidence.

We rely on the Therapeutic Goods Administration to ensure the basic safety of medications; trials and guidelines to give us overall direction and then we rely on the experiences we have. We rely on the universities, hospitals and colleges to put out qualified, competent specialists and then we just try them out to see what happens. Mostly, it will work out ok – and that's what you need to convince your patients.

CHAPTER 58

Tongue Lashing

If you've read this far, I trust you are enjoying both the content of this book, and hopefully the style. Words matter a great deal to me. (We asked for a hard copy of the Oxford English Dictionary as a wedding gift – I wanted the Complete but my wife won out with just the Concise).

Words matter to everyone.

Whilst it's hard enough to fit in history, examination, management plan and explanation all into one consult, it's also necessary to check that the patient properly understood what you said. Patients are nervous when they enter our consulting room, even if they've been seeing us for years (white-coat hypertension is proof of that!) and if it's a complex problem with a complex plan dealing with a condition unfamiliar to the patient and with potentially serious consequences, it is certain that not everything has been absorbed.

The counsel of perfection is to ask the patient to explain back to you everything they have understood. It isn't realistic to do that every time, but it's absolutely necessary to do that some of the time. Here's why:

A few years ago I did a telehealth consultation with a patient who normally sees another GP at our clinic. After dealing with his URTI I asked if there was anything else he wanted.

He said, 'No, not really – I'm just waiting for my heart to give out ...' This didn't make sense, so I asked what he meant. He replied, 'The cardiologist told me last time "There's nothing more I can do for you".'

As this was a patient I didn't know well, I had glanced through the file before calling him. I had noted a letter from the specialist which basically said "There's nothing else that needs to be done at this time – his angina is well-controlled and he is pain free".

This of course opened a whole other consultation! It transpired that he had spent the past 18 months depressed and expecting to die. He had quit his job and was just waiting ...

I explained the difference between "nothing that can be done" and "nothing that needs to be done", and at last report he had returned to his old profession and seemed much happier.

One might have hoped for a bit more self-reflection from the cardiologist involved when I told him this story. Though he didn't, let us at least learn something from this case in an effort to avoid making a similar mistake ourselves.

Our words cut.

And just as a scalpel can cure or can wound, so can our words. We can do a lot of healing with how we speak to a patient, and even more easily, we can do a great deal of harm.

CHAPTER 59

Compass Points

Over the next thirty or forty years of your clinical life there will be times when you will be tempted to become cynical. Don't! Please, don't!

You will be told that you are over-prescribing whilst being accused of ignoring patients' needs; over-investigating but being dismissive of patients with vague symptoms. You'll be told that you have the hardest job in medicine, but that you fail to keep up to date. You will be given guideline after guideline each of which will be presented as definitively best-care, and each of which will be superseded within years, months or (looking at you, PSA) every few weeks.

You will be progressively disempowered by regulation, expectation and imposition whilst roles that were clearly our domain are incrementally allocated to others with less training.

You will be told that you are the most cost-effective part of the health care system whilst being told that you are providing low level care too expensively.

Mostly you will be told this by people who have never worked in general practice, and many of whom have never spent a day sitting with a GP to see what we do.

Health economists have an important role to play in the system. There is a finite amount of money available. It needs to be rationally allocated. Their role is to determine where that should be.

The problem arises when they expect us to do their job for them. Despite all the obstacles thrown at GPs to prevent us doing our job freely, we are often told that GPs are why the Australian health care system is so efficient and so well regarded by others around the world. We are expert generalists who can carefully manage most acute disease, chronic illness and preventative health, and save the specialists, hospitals and expensive machines for those who really need them.

It is true that we are able to do that due to our knowledge, training and philosophy. But

We are guides more than gatekeepers.

We have obligations to patients, to families and to communities – but in that order. We should never (well perhaps better to say unbelievably rarely) compromise what is best for the patient sitting in front of us in the interests of an econocrat in Canberra.

That is not to say we should lie. If there are restrictions on a medication under the Pharmaceutical Benefits Scheme for only certain indications, then it is our obligation to comply. You can always offer a private script to circumvent funding restrictions. You may be surprised by how many patients – even on pension cards or Centrelink benefits – might be willing to pay for private medications, or even self-fund a specialist and private hospital care without any insurance cover.

Over the course of a career with individual patients – and their families – and a particular practice in a specific community – the greatest currency you have, the greatest power you hold, the greatest influence that you can apply – is trust.

A gatekeeper blocks entry. A guide shows you the front door, the back door and can even lend a hand to boost you through the window. I've never yet met anyone who extended their trust to a gatekeeper.

CHAPTER 60

Show Me Your Friends And I'll Tell You Who You Are

I had the pleasure of spending three years as a resident at Frankston hospital, which is now an outer suburb of Melbourne, but at that time almost a country town. It was run as a fee-for-service hospital where the specialists were all consultants with local private practices.

It didn't take long for me to develop my own favourites amongst the consultants. It was clear that some specialists were better than others – clinically more knowledgeable, surgically more skilled, kinder to their residents, and more engaging, caring and personable with patients.

Indeed, the great mystery to me was how some specialists survived in private practice at all. Frankston was a self-contained district, with maybe 100 GPs and 50 specialists. The specialists relied on the local GPs for referrals – and the local GPs rarely referred into the big city.

One of my first rotations was a mixed urology/psychiatry/gynaecology term. (It was a small hospital – they had to fill in the rosters!). Getting to know the specialists, I soon wondered why anyone would send a woman to gynaecologist A, B or C, when they could choose to send her to Drs D or E, who were clearly both better surgeons and nicer people.

I stayed in the Frankston area for several years and in multiple rotations. I noted the same pattern across most specialities. I also did several GP rotations in the area as a trainee, locum and eventually as an "assistant" – essentially a GP employee.

With time I realised that good GPs generally refer to good specialists. And working in several GP clinics in the same area led me to realise that good patients generally attend good GPs.

It took more time (and perhaps more maturity) to realise that by "good" specialists, "good" GPs and "good" patients, I actually meant specialists I liked, GPs like me and patients who liked me and whom I liked.

In other words

Patients select GPs who suit them; GPs select specialists who suit them.

It isn't so much a function of quality – though that is certainly one of the factors. Rather it's about good fit in style, preferences and priorities. Two surgeons might be equally skilled, but one more inclined to operate early; the other to wait and see. Both approaches may be reasonable. As a GP you should have your own thoughts based not just on the clinical picture, but your knowledge of the patient's values. Part of our GP role is to match the right patient with the right specialist for the right reasons.

Our patients are diverse in character and preferences. Since bedside manner and confidence are all critical parts of a therapeutic relationship, it makes sense that patients gravitate (where choice is available) to GPs who meet their needs. And it makes sense that if a patient chose a family doctor because they align with their values, that those are the same characteristics those GPs seek out in the specialists they refer to as they develop an address book from the multiple choices that they have.

The question then arises – if not all patients will love you, because you just won't suit everybody – do you need to try? At what point can you implicitly or even explicitly make it easier on yourself and your patient to move them on to another GP who might suit their values or preferences better?

I think that's a vexed question. There are GPs who make themselves doormats to be walked over by assertive patients, and compromise their own ethics, values, or even laws in order to try to please a patient who is only interested in their own desired outcomes – not in their best health interests.

There are also GPs who have an ego inflation that says they are under no obligation to adapt in any way to accommodate a patient's level of understanding, language, style or worries. An attitude which openly or implicitly says "My books are full. I have no interest or need to respond to your concerns."

Of course, the truth lies somewhere in between. You don't have to be all things to all patients. But I think the hallmark of professionalism is to try to subjugate your ego for the welfare of the patient .

CHAPTER 61

The One Beats The Many

We've already discussed in Chapter 24 that Evidence-Based Medicine (EBM) is science without a soul.

The process of developing knowledge is iterative and eternal. We know that we will never know everything about biology, disease, health and cure. If that is true about every individual aspect of medicine, it's even more true about medicine as a whole. In particular, about people.

Basic research studies and clinical trials are great at telling you what is statistically correct. They can give normal reference ranges, describe what 95% or 99.7% of the population are likely to do or how they are likely to respond.

But they are not great at telling you what applies to the complicated creature consulting you with his own preferences, desires, fears and history.

Evidence-Based Medicine tells you what is best for a thousand patients – but not for the person in front of you.

When I say "not", it suggests that EBM has no value for the patient you are consulting. Patently that isn't true. The evidence can tell you what is likely to work. Good research – a well thought out question, a well designed trial, a clear cut result, a solid but not overreaching recommendation – helps us provide the best care.

Yet we know the best care isn't always as effective as the journal said it would be. Is that because there are statistical outliers from the normal? Is it because our knowledge is not yet refined enough to understand genomics or gut flora or mind-body medicine, and once we master those unknowns our models will be more accurate? Is it because chaos theory teaches us that in a complex system (and what is more complex than people?!) nothing is ever entirely predictable?

All of the above, and probably more.

Being informed by the **science** means we have a base from which to work. Understanding the **patient** in front of us informs what is the right thing to do (or refrain from doing) for that person, at that time. It takes into account the complexity of his life.

Consider a 52-year-old man with a single episode of PR bleeding and no other symptoms. Would you recommend a colonoscopy, or would you suggest it is ok to wait a few months and see what happens? What would the guidelines say?

Now what if that man cared at home for a disabled adult child, and his wife was in palliative care with a life expectancy of a few weeks? Would that change what's published in the guidelines? Would it change your recommendation – or at least how strongly you pushed a particular course of action?

The motto of the RACGP is *cum scientia caritas*, formally translated as "with skill, tender loving care", but often roughly rendered as "knowledge with compassion".

There are two ways to parse "knowledge with care". One is that we should apply our knowledge and our care for our patients in equal measure, that either one without the other is of no value.

The other interpretation is that we should take care in applying our knowledge. Research is only as good as the question that it asks. Clinical thinking relies on knowing what research is relevant to this patient. Guidelines, evidence and algorithms are important for us – but not to them.

CHAPTER 62

Me, You, Us, Them

We have many roles as GPs. Some are plain, some less obvious and some seem to have been thrust upon us as a backhanded compliment. It's lovely that we are a profession in whom the public places sufficient faith to witness passport photos or certificates that require no medical training. But it isn't clear that it is the best use of our time.

We've noted that as GPs we treat patients, their families and the community. The latter is an interesting concept that seems to have evolved over time. Most GPs are not public health physicians (though many public health physicians did start as GPs). The days when GPs provided council immunisation services are long gone and the Doctors In Schools program struggles to get applicants.

Yet our GP forebears have served admirably in public health roles. Edward Jenner developed immunisation against smallpox, John Snow discovered the cause and cure of public cholera outbreaks.

Today, apart from our obligations to the patients who consult us, we are given the role as the gatekeepers to the entire health system. Our training and experience aren't just for show!

We don't refer every patient to a specialist. We don't arrange pathology and radiology for every presentation. We don't prescribe the latest, newest most expensive medications just because they are available when something cheaper will do just as well.

Why not? Because we have a societal role to protect the public, not only from ill health, but from system collapse.

There is however a profound conflict here, which was drawn to my attention by the late Dr David Levine from Johns Hopkins hospital in Baltimore. In a brief but profoundly influential conversation he pointed out to me that

Personal medicine does not serve the public; Public health does not serve individuals.

It summarises what I had felt but not articulated. If the welfare of our patient is all that mattered to us, well yes, we would ask for a specialist opinion for every niggle, we might arrange MRI for every sprain or abdominal pain.

We don't because the overall health system would rapidly collapse if we didn't apply some sense of logic, rationing and perspective. Yet none of that is the concern of the patient with us. If they pay taxes as required, why can't they call on the public purse to satisfy their health care needs and health care wants? If they want a specialist's opinion on a sprained finger – is it our role or right to decline their request for a referral? Or even to discuss the merits of the request rather than just acquiesce?

In reverse, what if they can afford to pay for these things privately? If a patient wants an MRI weekly, despite a very clear diagnosis of tension headache, and they are prepared to pay for it – who are we to stop them? Is there anything wrong with a system that would allow patients to directly access specialist and tertiary care without any checks along the way, if they are prepared to pay whatever the market cost is?

This is not a book on politics or economics – though both those topics are of great interest to me, and should be to every citizen, let alone every GP. Debates about individual rights and liberties vs communal responsibilities, fairness vs equality vs equity, the nature of social contract, are beyond this book and certainly beyond my expertise. But not beyond your obligation to think about!

There is no doubt that patients suffer and probably die because society refuses to pay for the very best care possible. An econocrat somewhere in Canberra has determined how many tax dollars should be spent on health and how many on education, defence, the arts, social welfare and on paying other econocrats. A second expert – or "expert" – has determined whether the health dollars provided should be spent on general practice, funding hospitals, subsidising psychologists, paying for medications or researching medical advances.

It's easy to demand more health dollars for patient rebates, though much harder to tell a teacher that class sizes may need to increase to pay for that, or a single parent that the pension will be cut. We can argue about government waste or say that foreign corporations should pay more tax or call for defunding arts programs that have a particular bias or that defence spending should increase or decrease. Inevitably, someone with different agendas and priorities will argue back.

In the meantime, recognise that you have an obligation to place the health and welfare of the patient in front of you as your most important priority. And that when ordering referrals, tests and medications subsidised by society, you have an obligation to do so rationally, placing the sustainability of the healthcare system as your most important priority.

CHAPTER 63

The A(B)C Of GP

Dr Paul Nisselle is rightly a legend in the Australian medical community for his encyclopedic knowledge and accessible analysis of medicolegal risks. A phrase of his that I repeat to every registrar during job interviews is not to be afraid of being sued. "The problem is not that doctors are sued too often – the problem is that we are not sued often enough".

The implication is that some patients being unhappy or having a bad outcome is inevitable through the course of a career. If a formal complaint is received every ten years or so, and if being sued happens once or twice in a lifetime, then when it does happen, we take it very personally. Many doctors question whether they should even continue in their career after being sued, despite objectively there being nothing that their peers would have done differently.

On the other hand, in the USA, where doctors can expect a law-suit, or at least a threat to sue every year or two, there is nothing shocking or shameful when a lawyer's letter arrives. You toss it into the "send to my medical defence organisation" pile and move on. It isn't personal!

Nisselle's dictum has certainly helped me absorb that avoidance of being sued is not a sensible approach to practicing good medicine. As has been pointed out, far too often doctors who are sued aren't negligent, and doctors who are negligent aren't sued.

Another of Paul Nisselle's sayings – he attributes first hearing it in the 1970s from Dr Roy Palmer, former secretary of the Medical Protection Society – is that for a successful career in a general practice a doctor must demonstrate the "4 As - Affability, Availability, Affordability and ... oh yes, Ability".

By the time I heard that saying, I had already developed my own, decidedly similar list. To be a successful and useful GP you need patients. And in choosing a GP, patients look for

The 5 Cs - confidence, competence, convenience, continuity and cost.

Confidence – your bedside manner. How comfortable are they that you know what you are doing and that you care enough to do the right thing by them rather than for yourself.

Competence – your skills. What are your outcomes? Do they get better? Are the scars you leave unsightly? Are the side-effects you generate acceptable?

Convenience – when is your clinic open? What services does it offer? How easy is it to get to by foot, car or public transport?

Continuity – when are you there? Are you available full time or part time, and are you available during the office and after-hours that are suitable for your patient's life, not your life?

Cost – for as much as people say they prioritise their health, the cost of general practice visits rarely figures when most people plan their household budget. They see us too infrequently, but for patients on limited incomes, a private fee consultation can be a big chunk of their free cash in any given week.

For a "health consumer", purchasing health services is no different to purchasing a TV or internet plans. They want the process to be easy, painless, cheap and perhaps to provide some degree of social cachet. It's only when things go wrong that people think more deeply about the consequences of their priorities. Both a used car and a new one will get you from here to there. You might prefer the features of the newer model, or you might prefer (or require) the savings of the older one. But when the car starts to break down regularly, you feel the cost of buying the cheaper option.

Similarly, most GPs in private billing clinics located near bulk-billing clinics will tell stories of how patients start coming when they feel the quality of care they seek outweighs the cost imposition. Whether true or not – and it's certainly not always true – they will perceive that paying extra results in better care.

Whether you choose to bulk bill or privately bill, and whether you choose the 4As or the 5Cs, your patient base and livelihood depends on the factors that matter to patients.

CHAPTER 64

Look It Up

When we first applied to become a teaching practice, we had to fill in lots of forms about why we wanted to take on the supervisor role, our facilities, demographics and so on. The RACGP put out a call for Expressions of Interest, and about 140 practices applied, but only around 20 were short-listed, so we were pleased to make that cut.

We then had a visit from an assessment team for an interview – perhaps oral exam is more accurate. One of the questions that we were asked was about our teaching experience. There are, I suppose, three ways to deal with oral exam questions – to give the standard, expected answer; to give a lengthy discourse that shows your deep knowledge of the topic (and allows you to chew up time that examiners might prefer to spend asking you questions you know less about); or to give an unexpected answer that shows a fresh approach with some greater insight. That way is a high-risk, high-reward strategy that might deeply impress and set an expectation that you exceed the base level required for all questions. Of course, if your answer isn't appreciated, then you come across as a smart-alec who is dodging the issue, probably because you don't know.

So when we were asked about teaching experiences, I could have replied referring to years of youth group work, my job whilst a uni-student teaching language on Sunday mornings, or the number of medical and pharmacy students we had already taken in to the practice. Instead, I went for the high-risk strategy.

"What do you mean? I teach every single day!"

I was looked at quizzically. So I reached for the dictionary on my bookshelf, turned to the appropriate page and quoted "'Doctor: From the Latin, meaning teacher.' Every time we see a patient, we explain what we are thinking, what is wrong, what we are going to do about it. We teach patients about how to use their puffers, how to take medications. We teach them preventative health strategies, physiology and anatomy, natural history and pharmacology."

Being a doctor means being a teacher.

Fortunately, or I would have missed out on 25 years of joy as a registrar supervisor, my response resonated with the panel.

There is debate in the general practice training world whether supervisors should be called by that title, or mentors, tutors, trainers, seniors, medical educators or some other term. I would be happy if we were just called teachers.

If you think back to the most memorable, impressive teachers you've had from kindergarten onwards, they were probably the ones who inspired you to love their subject, to love learning and to be better. They didn't just robotically recite the same words to every student who came through their class year after year; they made you feel like they were speaking to you in a way that you would understand. Yes, they may have set high standards and expectations; may have asked you to do things that made you initially feel uncomfortable. But because you felt that they genuinely cared for you and the subject at hand, you rose to the challenge they set. If they asked you to do something for which there may not have been an obvious reason at first, you complied because you trusted them.

In other words, your great teachers were great doctors.

I hope that you have the fortune, as I did, to stumble across an inspiring teacher, supervisor, mentor etc who will help shape you into a wonderful GP. (Thank-you Simmo!) I hope in turn that you take on the same role for the generations that follow. Indeed, one of the obligations in the original Hippocratic Oath is to teach the children of your teachers without fee or reward.

But mostly I hope that you become a great doctor – and therefore teacher – to your patients. You will need to listen carefully, explain thoroughly, work collaboratively, adapt to your patients' particular knowledge and values, have an engaging bedside manner, both genuinely care and show that you care, have patience and keep learning yourself.

CHAPTER 65

Know Their Why

Sometimes it's easy. The patient comes in, explains what they want, you provide a service, write your notes, send them out the door.

But often it isn't clear. A patient presents with vague symptoms. Or a vague history. Or without any clear agenda at all.

For ***bad*** GPs this can be a blessing. If the patient doesn't know what they want, how can the GP be expected to? So they do the minimum, the patient is out the door, usually without protest. Since they don't know what they want, how can they complain that the GP didn't provide it! And the GP can move on, satisfied that they have done all that was necessary.

A ***good*** GP will dig deeper and ask the patient to clarify, to ask if there is anything else going on, what else is bothering them and what they think might be the cause or cure.

But a ***great*** GP will ask a question of themselves.

What is the point of this consultation?

It is easier for a patient not to come to the doctor than to come. It costs time, money, effort to make an appointment, show up and be seen. If the patient isn't forthcoming on why they are there, you need to peel back what has motivated them to come to you, at this time.

In Chapter 31 we discussed the need to think about the timing of every consultation. Ask yourself – and if needed, ask the patient - Why is this patient here today – not yesterday, not next week? What are they asking for – diagnosis, treatment, medical certificate, cure, just an ear? Do they want to know what is wrong, or want to be told that nothing is wrong?

I remember when I was an intern that I had a cough which wouldn't resolve. After several weeks I went to my GP, Dr Les Segal (see Chapter 25) to complain, without any expectation that anything would or could be done. When he suggested an x-ray I shrugged him off, saying "It's probably 'just a cough'".

His reply has stuck with me. "It isn't just a cough. It's bad enough for you to have come in." (And of course he was right – it turned out I had mycoplasma pneumonia).

Les identified that when a patient walks through the door there is a reason, even if they don't know what it is. Probably it is population bias, but whenever I have a middle-aged man come in "just for a checkup", I am much more interested in the motivation for the visit than in the visit itself. Sometimes he comes in because his mate was just diagnosed with prostate cancer. Sometimes he has reached the age his father was when he died.

Sometimes it's to stop his wife nagging him to go see the doctor. In which case – what is her motivation? If he won't tell you – it's useful to just call her then and there. She may voice her exasperation – "Hasn't he told you about how he snores and then stops breathing? Or the weight gain? Or his drinking? Or his depression?"

Understanding the point of the consultation helps you identify not just why your patient is there, but also who the patient is!

Don't however fall into the trap of thinking there is only ever just ONE point to the consultation. It's too easy to have an "Aha" moment and stop looking further. Like foreign bodies in wounds, don't assume that there is only one.

Efficiently identifying the fundamental reason for a consultation is almost magical. Your patients will feel you are a mind reader or can see into the depths of their soul. You will feel like a master of your craft. And real health – not just treatment of illness – will be several steps closer.

CHAPTER 66

On Being A Real GP

More than 15 years ago, when I served as Supervisor Liaison Officer, I was expected to write a column every month or two for the Training Provider's newsletter. I think the following, lightly edited, is the one of which I am most proud.

~~~

I have recently celebrated my 15th anniversary in the same practice. Apart from pondering on the long-service leave that I would be entitled to in most other settings, but which seems mysteriously absent from my life as a practice principal, it has also been an opportunity to reflect on my concept of being a GP.

During my first term in general practice as a Family Medicine Program trainee I spent three months learning about Medicare item numbers, the PBS rules and the management of common presentations. They had to be awfully common presentations because in the space of a three-month term nothing that was uncommon presented often enough for me to recognise or review.

Nevertheless, that taste of general practice was enough to set me on my career path and, in my brash naivety, think that I knew what family medicine was about.

Fortunately, though I left the practice to do a term of geriatrics, I was asked to come back two or three nights a week to do a few hours helping out during the winter rush. I got to see a few families more than once; started to even recognise a few faces and names, and felt that now I had a true understanding of what being a (real) GP would entail.

Fast forward past a few more hospital terms, another couple of two- and three-month general practice stints and a trip overseas. I returned to my "home practice" to do what would now be called subsequent training. I spent 15 months learning from wonderful role models and from tolerant patients. I even developed enough of a following of patients to make me think I could make it out in the world on my own. After a year in the
~~~

same practice, I felt now I really knew what being a (real) GP meant.

So I found a small group practice, and talked my way in. I spent a year getting back to the level of familiarity with the patients and neighbourhood that I had had in my previous iteration, and again felt the flush of confidence that now I was a real GP.

But a funny thing happened over the next few years. I started to put together parents and children. Family history became more than just a routine question – I could see patterns of illness repeat across the generations. And I could see how a child's illness impacted the parent's health, and how the disease of a parent affected the child.

After five years, I recognised how much more profound my appreciation for the depth of general practice was. This, I thought, is what it means to be a real family doctor.

Another five years passed. Families moved in, grew and some moved out. Relationships formed and split up. Gradually a new set of connections fell into focus. I recognised adult siblings with different surnames, but with the same matriarch (rarely, upon reflection, was it a patriarch). Illnesses, patterns of behaviour, similarly dysfunctional families spread across three or four generations and with multiple branches. Watching children grow up and turn physically, emotionally and behaviourally into their cousins, their aunts and uncles, their grandparents. I heard both sides of marital breakdowns; sympathised with both the Hatfields and the McCoys.

The connection between individual and family had long been clear to me. Now it was about the relationship between family and family; between family and community. At last, I pondered, this is the true meaning of being a real GP.

And now, after 15 years, I have a different view altogether. Being a GP is not about the length of time one works in a practice, or even how long one provides scripts and referrals for a family. All that is necessary, but far from sufficient.

You become a GP when a family suffers its second major health crisis. The first crisis is not enough – that is when they come not knowing who to turn to. But see a family through one calamity with skill and compassion and the nature of the relationship will change. Upon their second misfortune – real or perceived, but real enough to them – they will turn to you not in hope, but in confidence. "Our doctor will see us through again".

Thus does one become a GP – not merely through the passage of time, but through the passing of crises; one extended family at a time, until you build a practice of those whose lives you have touched at their most vulnerable moments. Then you can call yourself a Family Doctor.

That at least is my theory for now. Ask me again after I've done it for another five years.

~~~

And if you were to ask me now, after yet another 15 years I would make one change.

You become a family's GP when they suffer their second health crisis.

And a real GP, when your day is full of such families.

The genie of part-time general practice is well and truly out of the bottle and is, probably, never going back. It's not impossible to be a great GP whilst working less hours, but I think it is much harder. Some of the very best GPs I know work part-time, and I now only consult half-time myself, the rest of my week being spent on teaching and practice administration. But my gradual reduction in clinical hours has highlighted to me even more clearly the difficulty in being a real GP when you aren't available to your patients when they need you, only when it suits you. Yet this is an issue that is rarely discussed.

It's a loss for the community. Health outcomes are clearly better with continuity of care by the same doctor. It's much less clear whether the same benefits accrue just by going to the same practice. It's obviously a loss for patients. But it's also a loss for GPs, where the greatest reward comes from long term, deep relationships with patients. The more you are there, the more you see each other, the more everyone will gain. The sooner then you will be, and love being, a real GP.
~~~

CHAPTER 67

The Big Reveal

I'm a great believer that everything in life that is worth doing comes only with great effort. Building and maintaining close friendships, relationships with partners, raising children – all take serious commitment. Learning another language, mastering a musical instrument, training for a marathon all take time and hard work.

Being a good GP, let alone a great one, also takes effort. And the primary strain is that you must always be on your toes. You need to constantly think. (Chapter 51).

The routine chest exam will not reveal a murmur if you aren't thinking. The Cushingoid facies is only visible to the GP who looks around the waiting room ... and thinks. The implication of needing to see a gynaecologist for a woman who has suffered sexual abuse only arises if you think.

Every reader here is smart, well-educated and well trained. You know how to think and you know that you should. But general practice is hard and exhausting and demanding.

Nonetheless – think! Because general practice is exhilarating and uplifting and emboldening – if you think! The thrill of the diagnosis, the satisfaction of peeling back the layers of the consultation, the little tactics you bring out in a series of visits to achieve a long-term strategic aim with a complex or recalcitrant patient are all the result of thinking.

Don't outsource your thinking. Don't rely on guidelines – be guided by them. Don't send your patients to allied health practitioners – lend them. Don't defer to specialists – only refer. Because you are the only person who has the knowledge, training and above all relationship with a patient to see both the macro and micro, the big picture and the passing scenes.

And if you don't ... then you should!

There is a balance between having an internal confidence, portraying a certainty of control and yet never assuming you are infallibly right or know what you are doing. When you have no idea what is going on – stop and think. Whenever you are comfortable you know what to do in any given situation – stop and think.

And once you really have mastered most situations and most problems and most conditions – go and study more so that you realise how little you know and that once again you must go back to the beginning – and think.

What makes general practice hard is what makes it so rewarding. What makes it so rewarding is what makes it hard. To get into medicine you had to compete with the best and the brightest. Don't lose the skills that got you there.

At the end of the day, I cannot emphasise strongly enough – **This whole book is a fraud!**

I've reduced some of the skills and some of the art of general practice to a series of glib cliches and aphorisms. But what I really want you to do is read them, consider them, adapt them – and then ignore them. What has worked for me works for me – in my era, in my practice, with my patients. You have to work out for yourself what will work in the world to come, with the patients you see.

There are universal human truths. And there are always changing times.

The key thing young people get wrong is saying "This time is different." The key thing old people get wrong is saying "Nothing ever changes."

Read what I wrote. Hear what your supervisors say. Talk to your friends. Read widely. Listen to wise people. Then ignore all of it – and think!

Humans are a mystery, and we'll never fully understand them. Embrace that challenge every day, and in every consultation –

Think!

CHAPTER 68

The Final Word

In the preface I mentioned that after treating two, three and four generations of the same family in the same practice over thirty-three years, I sometimes call myself a Grand-Doctor. It's been a grand experience to develop those relationships with the individuals, families and community of my suburb and surrounds.

No doubt there will be times in your career when you will get frustrated or have doubts about whether you took the right path. At those moments, try this exercise. Write down your job description of the best job imaginable. It might look something like this:

- Intellectually fulfilling – infinitely variable, always challenging and stimulating, with a breadth that is enthralling yet the opportunity to focus on a variety of sub-fields.
- Multi-faceted with the need to engage with both left-brain and right-brain thinking, fast and slow thinking, long-term and short-term thinking, and tactical and strategic thinking.
- Endless opportunities for formal and informal ongoing education as student and as teacher.
- Economically rewarding, with guaranteed demand for your skills and an income which puts you in the top 1-2% of workers. The capacity to work for yourself, work for others or to start your own business.
- A socially beneficial role that garners well-earned respect.
- The likelihood of working with (mostly) nice colleagues who care about the things that matter to you, and (mostly) nice clients who will genuinely show appreciation for what you do.
- The certainty that when you come home and your family ask "What did you do today?" you will have the

ability to answer with something new and interesting every day.

- When you need to make a point with your teenage children or have awkward conversations that you know they just won't want to have, you can bring it up indirectly by reference to something you saw at work. (Even, once or twice, when you didn't really. They'll never know!)
- An entertaining and engaging close-up view of a reality-TV soap-opera, where you can follow the complex stories of individuals and families across generations in this most fascinating of shows called life.
- A career which keeps you humble by reminding you how complex the world is and how small the part you play in it is, yet emphasises how every small part really matters.
- A job where you know that every day and over the course of your career you have made the world a better place.

This job would come with the income of a stockbroker, the moral worth of a social worker and the intellectual stimulation of a judge.

True – the job will also come with excessive paperwork, bureaucracy, the stress of constant change and the knowledge that you can do real harm. You will have to deal with high standards that you set yourself, and unrealistic expectations set by others – perhaps vice versa. You will be frequently told what to do by those who have little or no knowledge of what is actually helpful or possible.

But the benefits of the job so outweigh those disadvantages that it remains one of the most sought-after jobs. For good reason. Could there be anything better – more rewarding in all senses of the word – than a career in general practice? I honestly don't think so.

To reflect on a career where you have done good for individuals, families and the community provides a sense of fulfilment that most people can never attain. We have worked hard to get here. But we are incredibly, unbelievably fortunate to be able to do it. Every day we are intimately involved in the most valuable and interesting aspects of the human condition. Because

Every patient you see is a lesson in much more than the malady from which he suffers.

~~~

I would like to conclude by mentioning Ashley. You might not know Ashley – though she went to a school not far from yours. He really wanted to get into medicine. In fact – and you don't know this because it wasn't published – they were the very, very, very top candidate throughout the country who just missed out on getting into the medical course.

If even one other person – maybe you – hadn't taken up a spot, Ashley would have become a doctor, a GP. She was passionate and smart and caring, but ever so slightly not at the level to get in. He would have been great – a dedicated clinician to patients, resource to colleagues, teacher to juniors and integral part of his local community. But due to the tiniest of shortfalls, they just didn't make it because every slot was filled.

If you had chosen another path, Ashley would now be a doctor – perhaps even in your practice, looking after your patients. And I think you owe her something - because his dream was stymied by your choices. Ashley would have worked long hours, been a complete GP, taught and served, been caring and skilled and driven to make a difference.

But Ashley isn't a GP. You are. And I think that comes with a responsibility – to be a better GP than Ashley would have been.

General practice is the best job in the world.

Never forget that. Always appreciate that.

I hope that you too experience the boundless satisfaction that comes from being a Grand-Doctor. I hope you love your life in general practice.

Enjoy.
~~~

Epilogue

Now I'm scared to send my patients to ED.

I know so much better than they do
who my patients are and what they need.

That once panic-stricken registrar,
twenty-five years later.

I desire no other epitaph ... than the statement that I taught ... as I regard this by far as the most useful and important work I have been called upon to do.

Dr William Osler, The Fixed Period, 1905

APPENDIX

Some Thoughts For Supervisors

- A GP builds relationships with patients by treating them with care, knowledge, respect and as individuals. A supervisor builds relationships with registrars the same way.
- Impress your registrar with your clinical acumen in the first two weeks, and they will trust you for the rest of the term.
- Never underestimate how much a registrar learns by observing rather than hearing.
- Sit-in tutes (watching a registrar consult) always reveal a teachable moment – something that has been done well and needs to be reinforced, or something that can be done better and needs to be worked on. Don't leave your registrar seeing your patients to a Medical Educator's External Clinical Teaching Visit.
- Be very sparing in running group tutes. You aren't teaching what to do, you're teaching how to think, and every registrar thinks differently.
- Better to teach a little bit often, than a lot infrequently.
- Registrars only ever ask three questions – What's the diagnosis? What's the treatment? Am I doing ok? Rarely answer the first. Sometimes answer the second. Always answer the third.
- Don't waste any opportunity to learn from and be inspired by your registrar – they are colleagues, they are fresh and they know lots that we don't.
- The in-practice training program is only two years long and not a day should be wasted. Every day, ask your registrar "What did you learn today?"

I feel a very unusual sensation –
if it's not indigestion,
I think it must be gratitude.

Benjamin Disraeli

Gratitudes

Writing a book is a marvellous way to appreciate how many good people you have in your life.

I must start with someone I barely know. Dr Patrick Kinsella heard me mention a few of these aphorisms in passing a decade ago, insisted that I present them at a supervisors' workshop and then repeatedly encouraged me to turn this into a book. He had vision before I did and his faith in the idea motivated mine. I am very grateful.

I have been inspired by many friends, local and international, who have written their own books, and I thank them for the "if they can do it – so can I" motivation.

I have been blessed by having wonderful teachers at all stages of my life, but first among equals is Dr John Siemienowicz and the team at Langpark Medical Centre who provided me with the formative experience of general practice that made me fall in love with the profession and provided the model of practice which I wished to emulate.

For over forty years, Dr Les Segal has been my GP, teacher, mentor, *veg-vayzer* and, above all, friend. He is the complete GP – kind, knowledgeable, caring, passionate, sensible. I also admit it – he's much funnier than me.

I have learned from a multitude of great GPs and specialists. I cite many of them in this book and thank them for what they taught me and for their consent to quote – Drs Peter Arnold, Grant Connoley, Peter Grossberg, Mary Jackson, the late David Levine, Richard McNeill, Paul Nisselle, Roy Palmer, Lindsay Quennell, Steven Scully and Les Segal. I have also used quotes that my notes attribute to Drs Tim Diamond and Clare Turner though I have not been able to locate and contact them to confirm. I ask forgiveness if that is in error.

Parkridge Medical Centre was established by Drs Wayne Piez and Glenda Ferguson, and nurtured by Drs Ray Carne, Mary Jackson and Peter Tribe. Wellness on Wellington would never have existed without them and I thank them for laying the foundations of my professional home.

The reception, nursing, GP, specialist and allied health team of Wellness on Wellington are a joy in my life. To spend most of my working life with a team of people who care for patients and for each other to such a level has been a boon and blessing. As an exemplar of dedication to care, hard work and focus on that which matters, I particularly want to thank Louise Trevean. She is, in all senses, WoW!

My never-complaining former registrars and now colleagues and work partners – Drs Kateena Vogel, Peter Yee and Joel Jaya – have long had the right to insist I speak less about the frustrations of writing the book and more about dealing with the needs of the practice. I am deeply grateful for their understanding of my visceral need to complete this text, and their constant support whilst I undertook it.

It's said we only need three friends. I am blessed to have had Benny, Leon and Joe supporting me in all parts of my life for five decades and more.

The book didn't write itself, and it certainly didn't get better by itself. Thank-you to those who read the first draft – Drs Zachary Berger, Kirrily Ellerton, Elana Forbes, Patrick Kinsella, William Kinsella and Harishan Tharmarajah. I am especially grateful for the detailed and thoughtful reflections, suggestions, corrections and comments that I received from Drs Simon Craig, Ross Lomazov, Josh Osowicki, Ron Roth and Les Segal.

The second draft was read by Drs Chris Dickie, Srishti Dutta, Priya Maheson and Professor Karen Price. I appreciate their kind comments and useful suggestions. Dr Ken Sikaris provided valuable feedback on Chapter 14.

You can't judge a book by its cover, but you can judge the cover by its quality. Monique Bendel has been enthusiastic, creative, knowledgeable and a great pleasure to work with on the cover design.

General practice is better termed family medicine, not only because we treat families, but because our families inevitably become enmeshed in our professional lives. I thank Ruth, Yoni, Hillel and Aydl for tolerating my career despite the significant impact on them, and for accepting even less time with me whilst I wrote this work. I deeply hope that my children derive as much satisfaction from both their careers and their children as I have from mine.

Any spelling, grammar or punctuation errors are entirely Ruth's fault for not picking them up after multiple rounds of proof reading and editing. I appreciate her efforts anyway. I appreciate pretty much everything else about her as well.

Penultimately – I want to thank the nearly 100 registrars that I have taught. I developed these rules from you and for you. You have been an inspiration in all ways possible and kept me practicing when I might otherwise long have retired. Above all, you have taught me far more than I have taught you.

And lastly, I wish to thank my patients who have made thirty-five years in general practice the most satisfying career possible. This book is largely based on the lessons I have learned from the mistakes that I have made and that you have suffered. Though I always had your best interests at heart, I am very aware of how often I fell short. I extend my deepest thanks to you for trusting that I knew what I was doing.

Summary

1. You have to deal with the patient's agenda before you deal with your own.
2. Your primary duty at any consultation is to get another one.
3. In General Practice, every patient has a name.
4. What does the patient want? What does the patient need?
5. The patient wants to tell you their story!
6. Wash your hands after every examination – it gives you time to think.
7. Always put the patient on the couch.
8. At every consultation, a good GP does one thing the patient didn't ask for.
9. Investigations are merely a numeric or pictorial approximation of the patient's clinical condition
10. What we learned when we were young stays imprinted – rightly or wrongly.
11. If the history is unrevealing take more history.
12. If you don't know what it is, tell the patient what it's not.
13. If the patient doesn't mention cancer, MS, Alzheimer's, Parkinson's (or MND) – you must.
14. Fourteen tests equals an abnormality.
15. An emergency is when a patient changes shape or colour.
16. Always believe the patient – especially the mother.
17. Believe nothing that the patient tells you.
18. A child who is active enough to get into trouble is probably not in trouble.
19. It is not essential to have the answer, but it is critical to have a plan.
20. Steal time from the rich and give to the poor.
21. Sometimes for good and sometimes for bad – muttering kills silence.
22. Why do we review a patient?

23. You don't need to know every diagnosis. But you need to know that there are ones you don't know.
24. There is no evidence for Evidence-Based Medicine.
25. Go up to the patient in the waiting room.
26. More mistakes in medicine are made by not looking than not knowing, but most mistakes are made by not caring.
27. There are rarely sharks in swimming pools.
28. Every question must have a purpose.
29. If you are going to lose sleep over it, do something about it.
30. The doctor does the thinking; the patient does the feeling.
31. What came before? What comes after?
32. No ferritin or FBE is complete without looking at previous results.
33. Patients pay the doctor to do the worrying for them.
34. Patients hate spot diagnoses.
35. Sometimes you have to choose between comprehensive notes and a comprehensive consultation.
36. When you don't know – go back to university.
37. Normal does not always mean OK.
38. Never say the word "just". Never use a phrase with "quick".
39. When referring to a specialist – lend, don't send.
40. The most important line on a radiology report is the signature.
41. If you want to get the consultation over as quickly as possible – don't! When a consultation is going badly, stop the consultation and say, "This consultation is going badly."
42. Perfect is the enemy of Good; Good is the enemy of Perfect.
43. No diagnosis is complete without a differential diagnosis.
44. A consultation must be the 3 Es – effective, efficient and engaging.
45. Beware the last patient of the day; especially on a Friday; especially before a holiday.
46. The illness is the illness.
47. A consultation is a dance.
48. Be enthusiastic about telehealth. Be enthusiastic during telehealth.

49. Don't be confident till you've made mistakes.
50. A doctor who is offended by a request for a second opinion is someone whose primary opinion is not worth worrying about.
51. It's not that general practice is boring. It's that it lulls you into a false sense of serenity.
52. A good consultation may be a short case or a long case but never a series of short cases.
53. Specialists cut with a knife; GPs peel back layers.
54. After a prolonged absence, return to work on a Friday
55. Always recap the dipstick bottle before opening the urine jar.
56. The more a patient talks, the more you'll hear what they don't say.
57. If there are many treatments for a disease, none of them are any good.
58. Our words cut.
59. We are guides more than gatekeepers.
60. Patients select GPs who suit them; GPs select specialists who suit them.
61. Evidence-Based Medicine tells you what is best for a thousand patients – but not for the patient sitting in front of you.
62. Personal medicine does not serve the public; Public health does not serve individuals.
63. The 5 Cs - confidence, competence, convenience, continuity and cost.
64. Being a doctor means being a teacher.
65. What is the point of this consultation?
66. You become a family's GP when they suffer their second health crisis.
67. Think!
68. General practice is the best job in the world. Never forget that. Always appreciate that.

About The Author

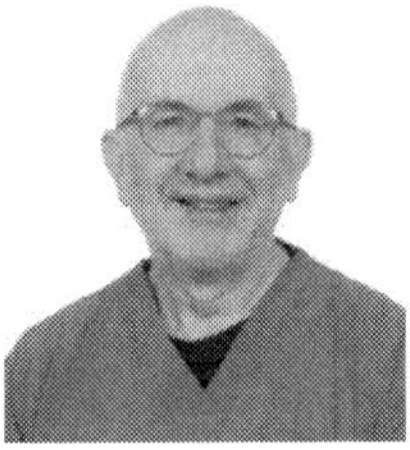

David Ringelblum has been a GP at Wellness on Wellington in Rowville, Melbourne for 33 years, treating up to four generations of families.

He is passionate about teaching GP trainees and is proud to have supervised nearly 100 registrars over the past thirty years, and even prouder that twenty are now his practice colleagues.

He has been nominated multiple times as Supervisor of the Year, winning the award in 2008; received the Outstanding Contribution award for the Victorian Metropolitan Alliance Regional Training Program in 2009, and led the clinic to win the EVGPT Teaching Practice of the Year award in 2022.

Under his leadership, Wellness on Wellington was also a Finalist in the AGPAL Chair Practice of the Year award in 2018.

David was an examiner for the FRACGP exam for over ten years; has spoken on behalf of the Knox Division of General Practice and Eastern Primary Health Care Network on public health issues; provided regular guest appearances on SBS radio and the 3RRR "Radiotherapy" program speaking on general practice matters and ethical issues; and been rebroadcast internationally as a health advisor.

Apart from practicing and teaching general practice he is passionate in equal measure about his family, community volunteer work, and chocolate.

Made in United States
Orlando, FL
04 November 2026

90201282R10120